Wellness Warriors

Written by
**Mort Greenberg &
Carly Greenberg**

Forward

Are you ready to embark on an extraordinary journey toward a healthier and more vibrant life? This book is your guide to unlocking the secrets of well-being, filled with insights and practical tips that will empower you to make positive choices and transform your lifestyle.

In the fast-paced world we live in it's easy to get caught up in the whirlwind of screens, stress, and unhealthy habits. But fear not! With each turn of the page, you'll discover a wealth of knowledge and wisdom that will help you to take charge of your well-being.

Throughout the next ten captivating chapters, you will be able to explore topics designed to enlighten and inspire. This book covers everything from the impact of screen time and the significance of posture to the wonders of physical activity, nutrition, mental health, and the importance of rest and recovery.

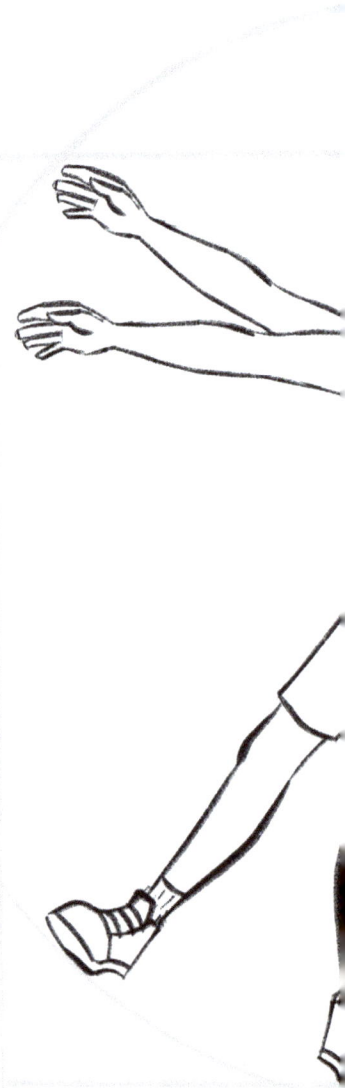

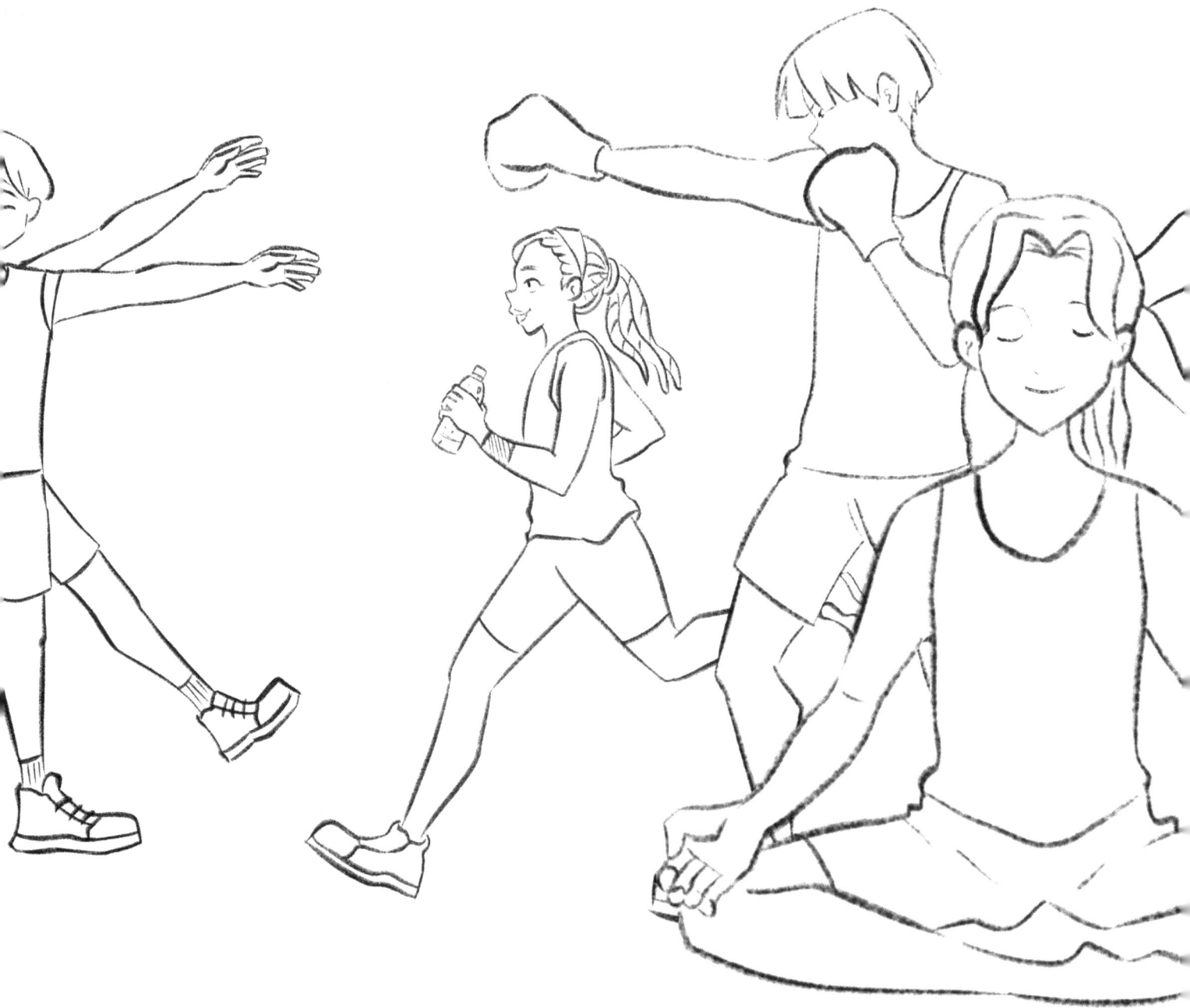

Copyright © 2023 by
Mort Greenberg & Carly Greenberg

Design: Heri Susanto
Illustrations: Dian Kartika Abidin

First Paperback edition December 2023

ISBN 978-1-961059-01-6 (Print)
ISBN 978-1-961059-03-0 (EPUB)
ISBN 978-1-961059-02-3 (Kindle)

Published by TuckEmIn
www.tuckemin.com

Introduction

Tuck Em' In Publishing is a father-and-daughter effort that creates and publishes books for kids. Our mission is to Motivate and Inspire. Our vision is to help kids make the most of their todays and tomorrows.

The Fearless Girl and The Little Guy with Greatness is a book series that aims to share the following message: anything is possible for any kid if they put their mind to it.

Kids, in our books, you can find ways to handle yourselves in critical, real-life situations. Caregivers, you will find ways to push the kids in your life to be their best selves. Through our books, we encourage families to communicate more effectively with each other.

"Wellness Warriors" is the sixth installment in The Fearless Girl and The Little Guy with Greatness book series. This book will move through 10 topics: 1) Screen Time and Digital Well-being, (2) Posture, (3) Warm-Ups, Cool Downs, and Physical Activity, (4) Martial Arts and Mobility, (5) Hydration, Electrolytes, and Limiting Sugary Drinks, (6) Balanced Diet, Mindful Eating, and Portion Control, (7) Healthy Snacking, Cooking, and Meal Preparation, (8) Dental Health, (9) Mental Health and (10) Rest and Recovery.

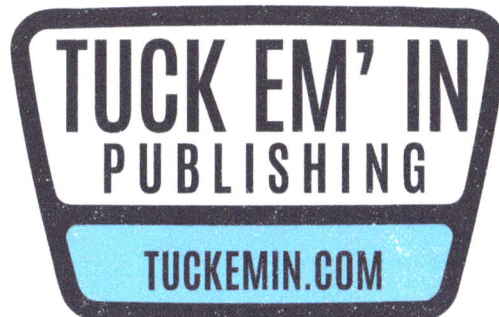

TUCK EM' IN PUBLISHING

TUCKEMIN.COM

Mort Greenberg and his daughter, **Carly Greenberg**, have embarked on numerous adventures together across the mountains of the United States. They also built self-guided, 18-hour day races in London, Paris, Milan, Venice, Murano, Burano, Rome, Buenos Aires, Tigre, Montevideo, Valparaiso, Santiago, Asuncion, and more.

This father and daughter team has worked through and overcome the same situations that you, as a parent, are experiencing now with a young daughter or son. Each skill in the book is inspired by an actual conversation that took place over the years from when Carly was five to twelve years old.

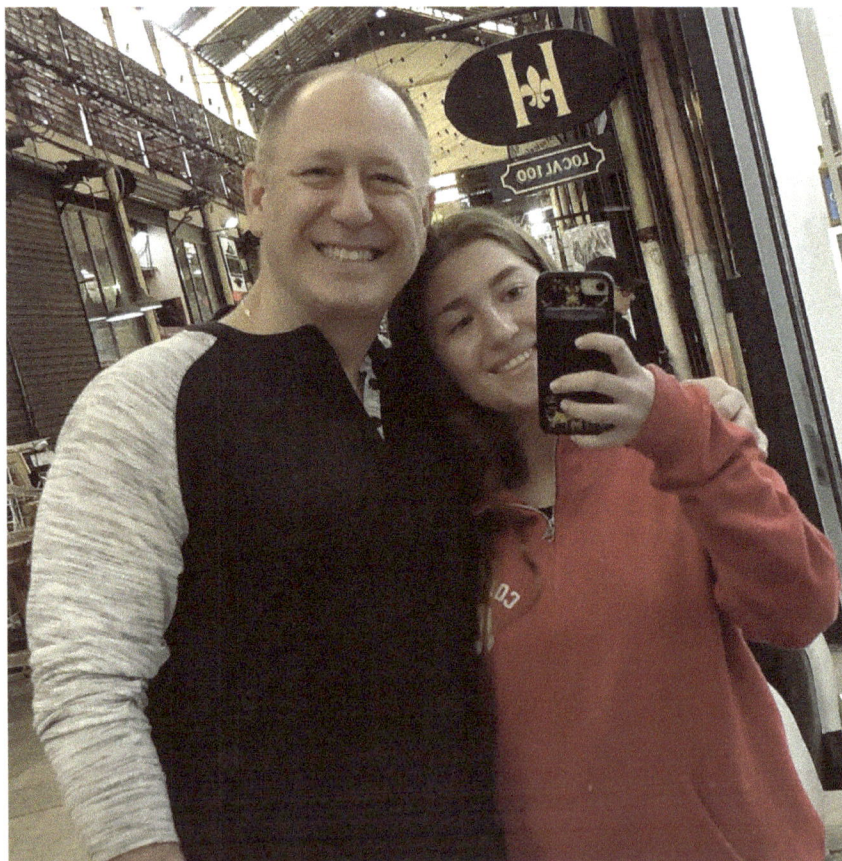

You Can Follow Mort and Carly on social media:

@mortgreenberg

@greenbergcarly

@mortgreenberg

@carlygreenberg

This Book Belongs to

_____

Today's Date : _____

Table of Contents

Chapter 6 : Balanced Diet, Mindful Eating, and Portion Control

Your body needs a balanced diet to be strong and energetic. You will learn about fruits, veggies, whole grains, proteins, and healthy fats. You will also discover mindful eating, which means savoring your meals and listening to your hunger and fullness cues. Oh, and portion control is essential, too, so that you don't overeat.

Chapter 7 : Healthy Snacking, Cooking, and Meal Preparation

Ready to be a kitchen whiz? You'll learn how to prepare delicious and healthy snacks. You'll even find a few simple recipes you can prepare with the help of adults. Cooking can be so much fun! You'll explore different cooking methods like baking, grilling, and steaming. Plus, you'll get involved in meal planning and preparation at home.

Chapter 8 : Dental Health

Caring for your teeth is vital for a healthy mouth and overall well-being. You'll learn about brushing your teeth at least twice daily, flossing, and visiting the dentist regularly. Always keep your pearly whites shining bright!

Chapter 9 : Mental Health

Did you know that your emotions affect your overall health? It's essential to take care of your mental well-being. You'll learn about expressing your feelings, seeking support from trusted adults, and doing activities that make you feel good.

Chapter 10 : Rest and Recovery

Did you know rest is as essential as being active? Your body needs proper rest and recovery to stay strong and avoid injuries. You'll learn why getting enough sleep and rest from intense activities allows your body to recover, repair muscles, and prevent overuse injuries.

Chapter 1

Screen Time
and Digital Well-Being

Are you ready to uncover the secrets of screen time and discover how it can affect your health? In this chapter, we'll dive into the world of screens and learn how to maintain a healthy balance between your digital devices and other exciting activities.

What You Need to Know

Did you know that spending too much time in front of screens can impact your body and mind? While screens can be awesome for learning and having fun, too much screen time can make you feel tired, affect your sleep, and even strain your eyes. To ensure you have a healthy relationship with your devices, it's important to limit how much time you spend with screens.

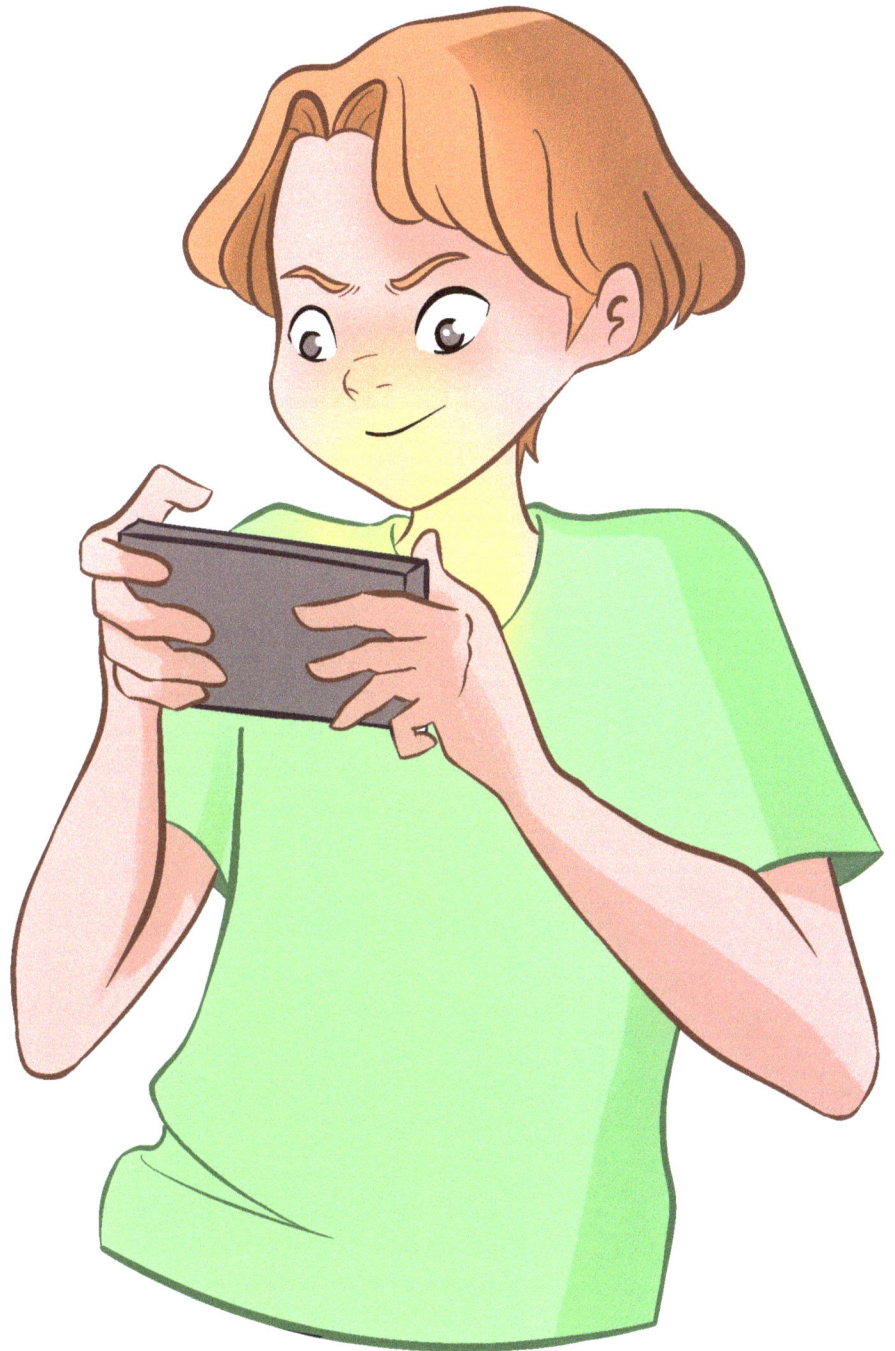

Try It Activities

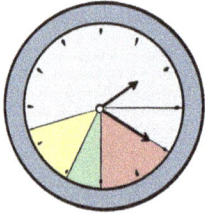

Build a Screen Time Schedule
Create a daily schedule that includes time for home-work, physical activity, hobbies, and screen time. Stick it on your wall, or use colorful stickers to make it fun and easy to follow.

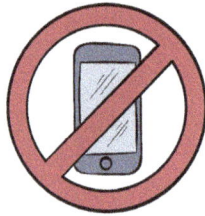

Device-Free Zones
Create spaces where screens are not allowed in your day and home. It could be during mealtime or in your bedroom before bedtime. This way, you can focus on connecting with your family or enjoying quiet time.

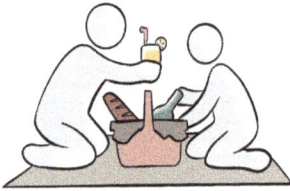

Screen-Free Challenge
Challenge yourself and your friends to go one whole day without screens. Plan activities like board games, building forts, or having a family picnic. Share your experiences and see who can create the most exciting screen-free adventure!

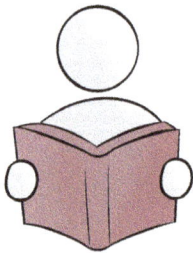

Bookworm Challenge
Set a goal to read a certain number of books each month. Make a cozy reading nook, get lost in mag-ical stories, and let your imagination soar. Reading expands your knowledge and gives your eyes a break from screens.

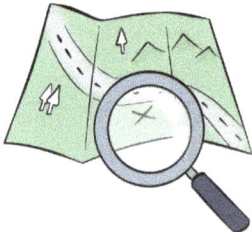

Tech-Free Treasure Hunt
Design a treasure hunt around your house or neigh-borhood using clues and riddles. Invite friends or fam-ily members to join in the fun. This interactive activity will keep you engaged and away from screens.

"

Remember, finding a healthy balance between screen time and other activities is the key to digital well-being. Limiting your screen time and exploring new adventures unlock endless growth, creativity, and fun possibilities.

Chapter 2

Posture

Have you ever wondered why sitting for a long time can affect your posture and health? Get ready to unlock the secrets of good posture and discover how it can make you feel amazing inside and out. In this chapter, you'll learn tips and tricks for sitting, standing, and using your devices with the best posture.

The Power of Good Posture

Did you know that good posture helps keep your body aligned, supports your muscles, and makes you feel confident and strong? When you slouch or hunch over, it can strain your muscles, lead to back pain, and even affect your breathing.

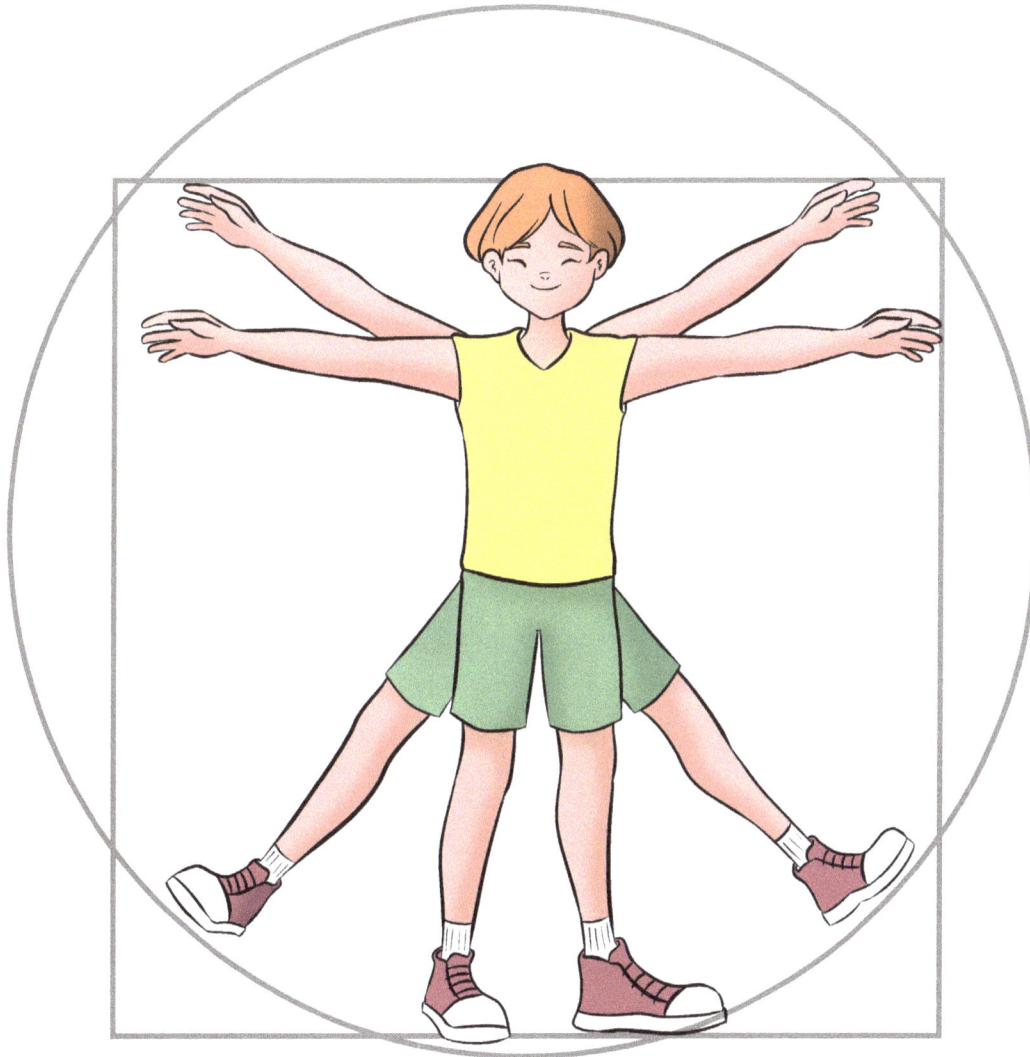

Tips for Sitting

Chair Magic

Choose a chair that allows your feet to touch the ground comfortably. Sit all the way back in the chair and keep your back straight. Imagine a string pulling you up from the top of your head, helping you sit tall.

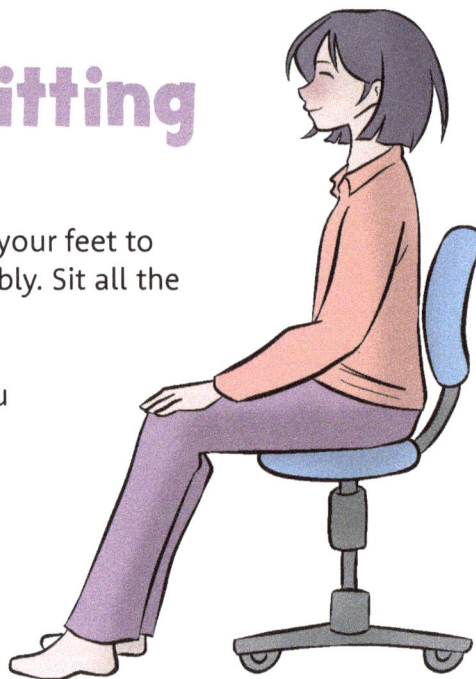

Active Sitting

These movements help keep your muscles active and prevent stiffness.

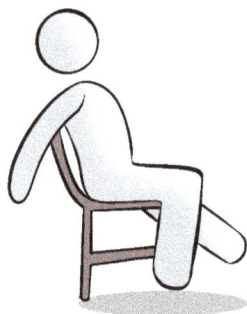

Wiggle and move while sitting

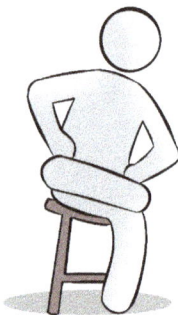

Shifting your weight from side to side

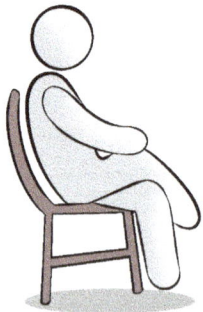

Crossing and un-crossing your legs

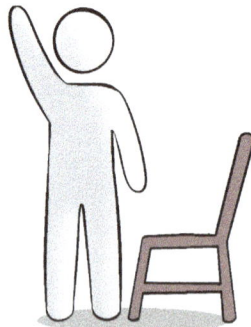

Taking short standing breaks

Stand Tall

Backpack Heroes

If you carry a backpack, adjust both shoulder straps so your bag sits snugly on your back. A balanced load helps prevent strain on your spine and promotes better posture.

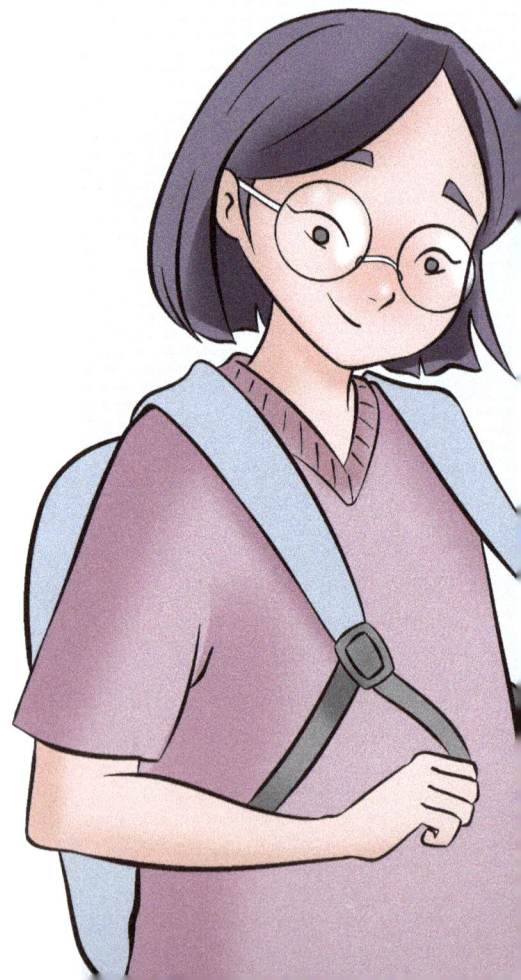

Stretch Breaks

Take short breaks from sitting or standing for long periods. Stretch your arms overhead, reach for the sky, and gently twist your upper body from side to side. These stretches keep your muscles flexible and happy.

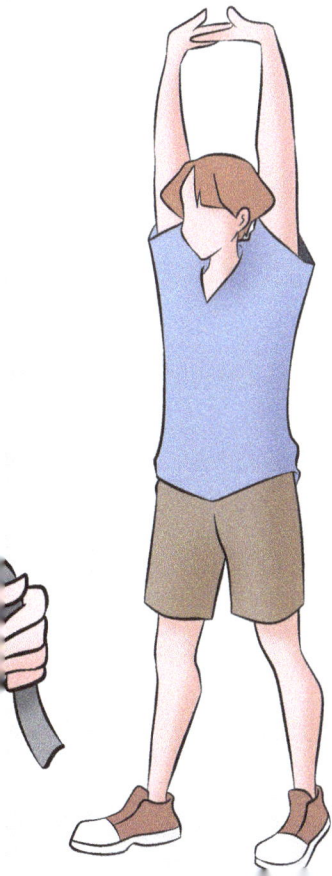

Device Dexterity

Smart Desk Space

Create a comfortable work-space by correctly setting up your desk and chair. Ensure your elbows are at a com-fortable 90-degree angle and your computer screen is directly in front of you, at eye level. This way, you can work comfortably without straining your neck or back.

Screen Eye Level

When using electronic devices, like tablets or phones, try to keep them at eye level. Avoid look-ing down too long, as it can strain your neck and shoulders. You can prop up your device or adjust the angle of your screen to achieve this.

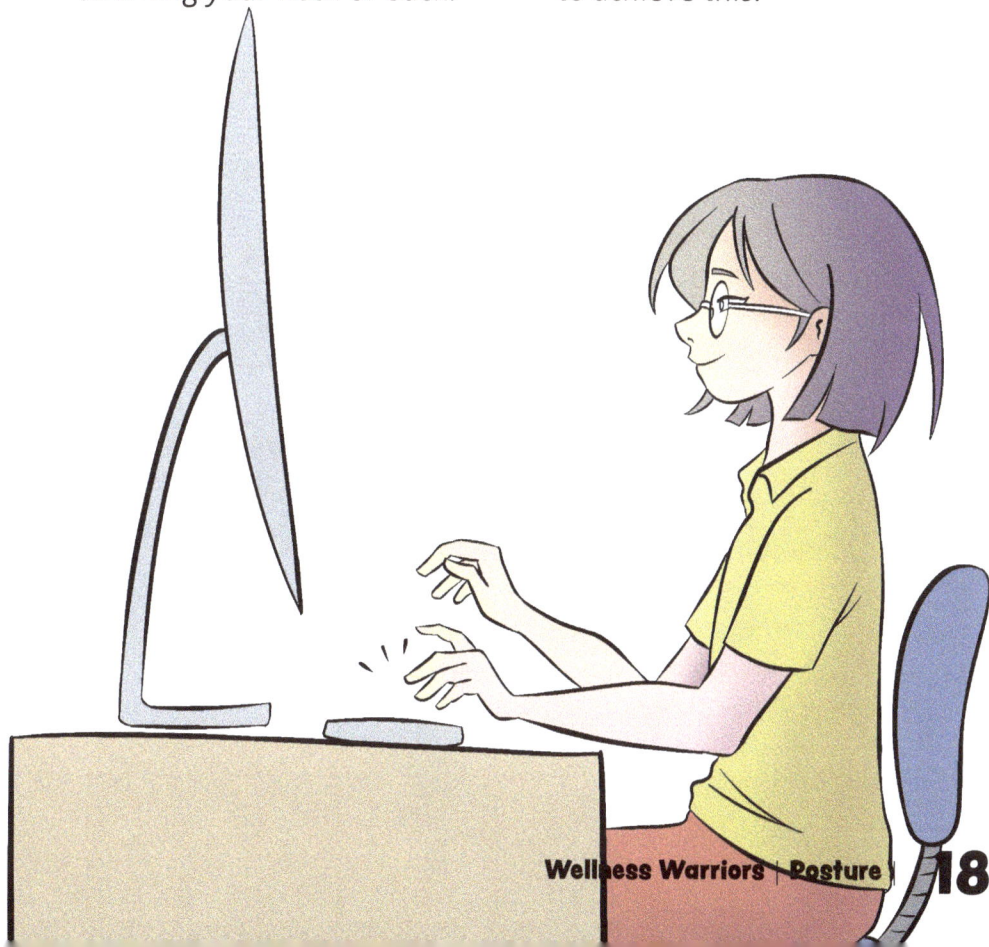

Try It Activities

Mirror Mirror

Stand in front of a mirror and practice standing tall with good posture. Imagine you're a superhero striking a confident pose. Hold it for a few seconds, repeat throughout the day, and watch your posture improve.

Balloon Breathing

Inhale deeply, expanding your belly like a balloon. As you exhale, imagine a string pulling your head upward, lengthening your spine. This exercise helps you engage your core and maintain good posture.

Puppet Strings

Pretend you're a marionette puppet with strings attached to your head, shoulders, and back. Imagine someone gently pulling the strings, lifting you up, and aligning your body. Walk around, feeling light and controlled.

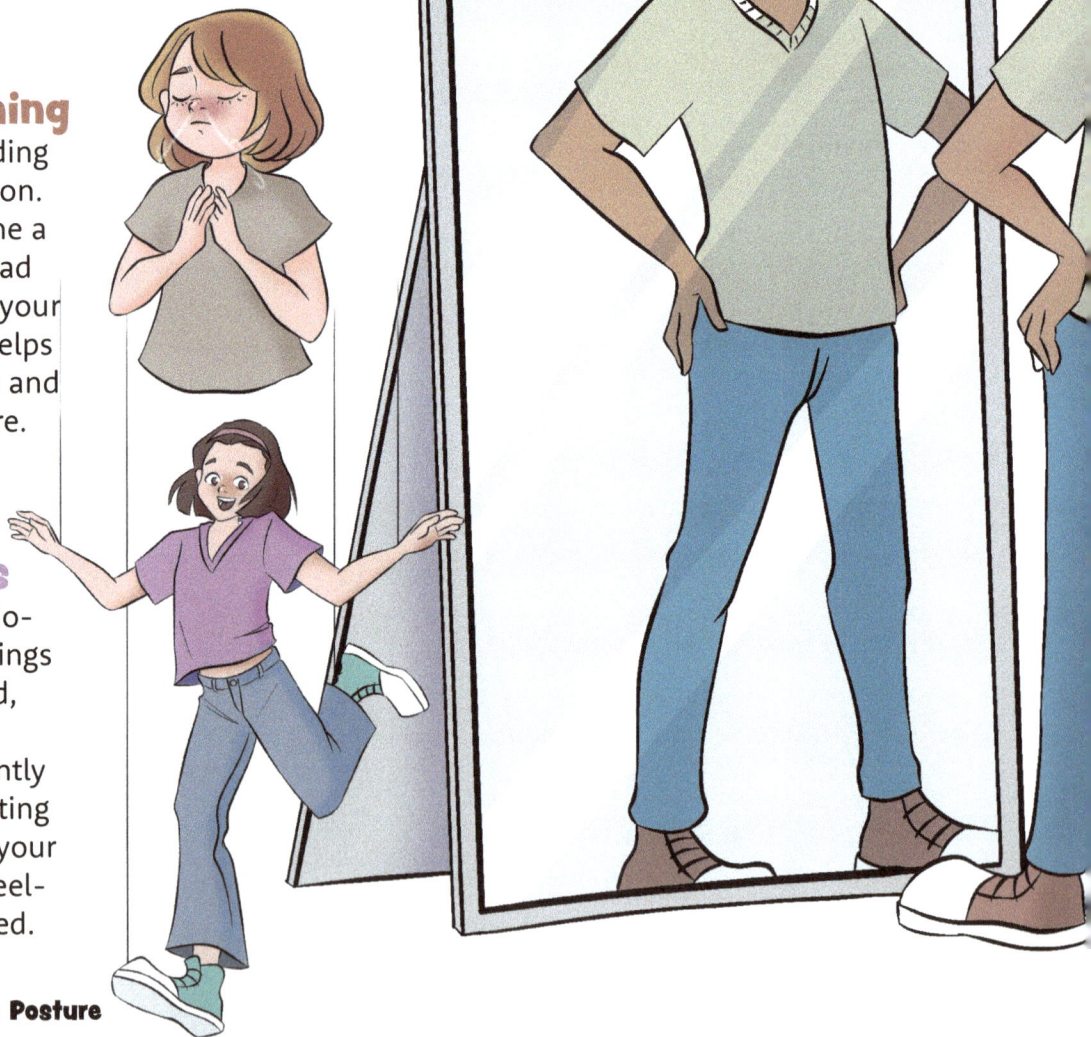

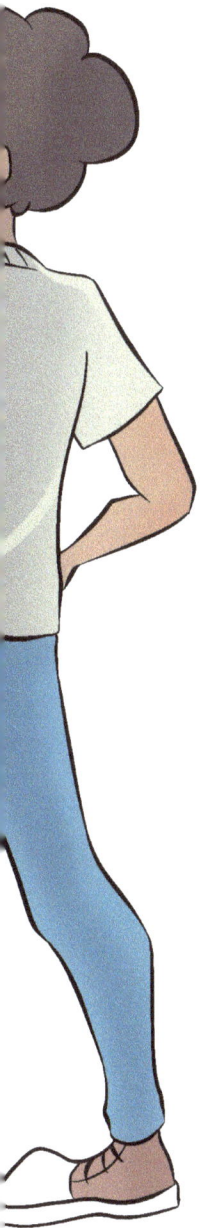

You'll become a posture superstar by incorporating these exercises and tips into your daily routine. So, stand tall and walk proud.

Chapter 3

Warm-Ups, Cool-Downs, and Physical Activity

Regular exercise is fun and important for your health and development. In this chapter, we'll focus on warming up and cooling down before you take on your sport of choice today, like biking, swimming, cross-training, weight lifting, bodyweight exercises, or being active outdoors.

The Power of Exercise

Exercise strengthens your muscles, improves your heart and lung health, boosts your energy, and even helps you feel happier. Being active is the key to a healthy and strong body.

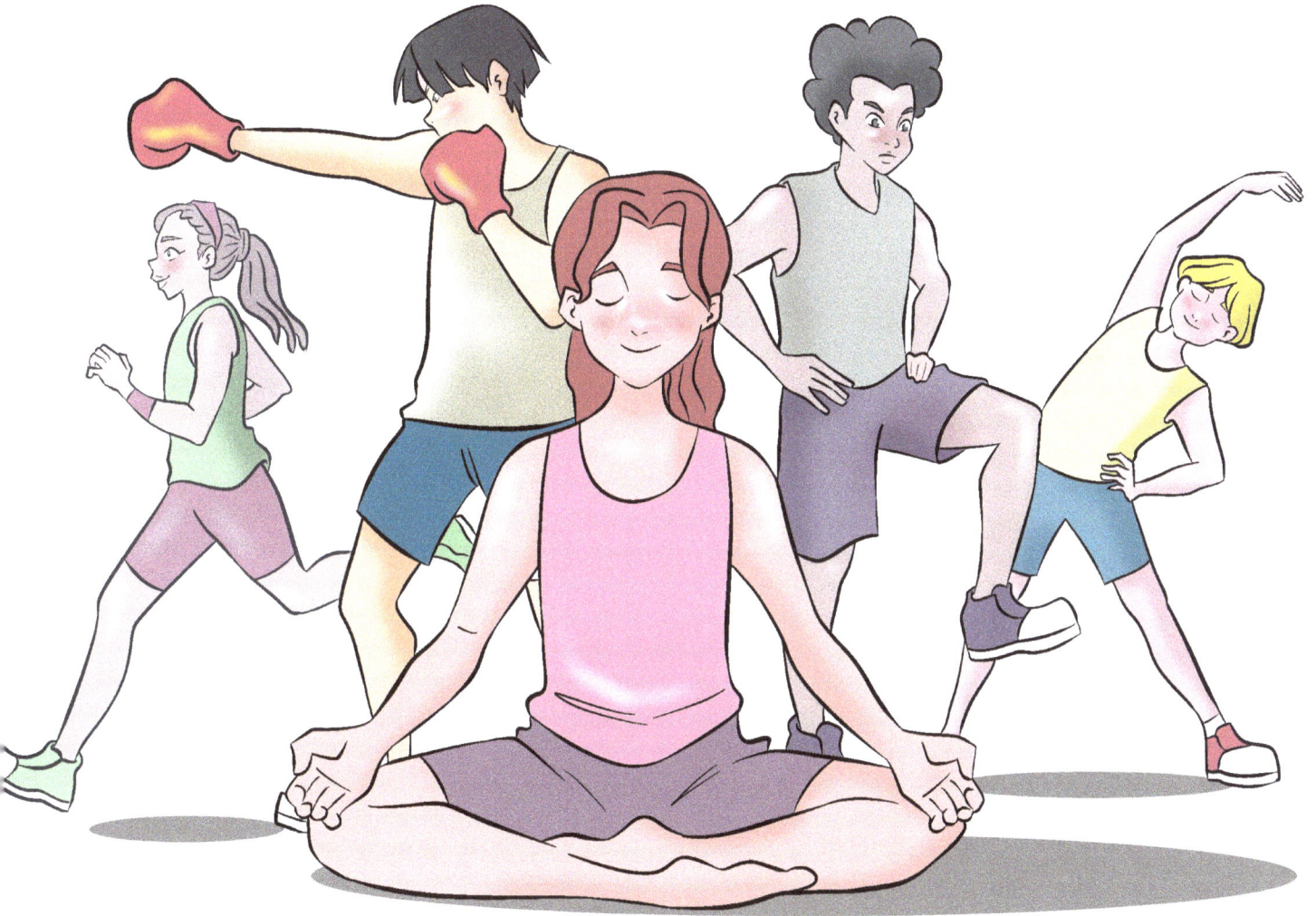

Warming Up

Before you start any physical activity, it's crucial to warm up your body. Warming up prepares your muscles and joints for action and helps prevent injuries. Here are some simple warm-up exercises to try:

Jumping Jacks

Stand with your feet together, then jump and spread your legs wide while raising your arms above your head. Jump back to the starting position and repeat. This exercise warms up your whole body.

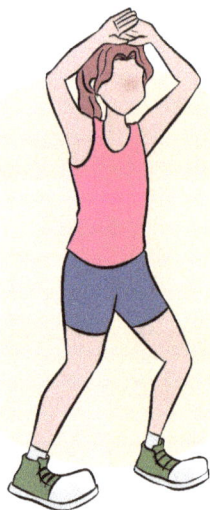

High Knees

Stand in place and lift your knees as high as possible, alternating between each leg. This exercise warms up your leg muscles and gets your heart pumping.

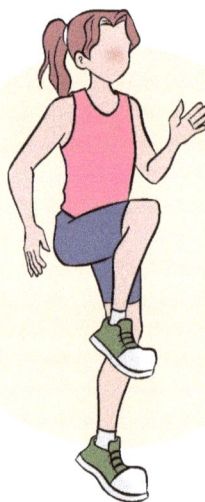

Arm Circles

Stand with your arms extended to the sides. Make small circles with your arms, gradually increasing the size. This exercise warms up your shoulder muscles.

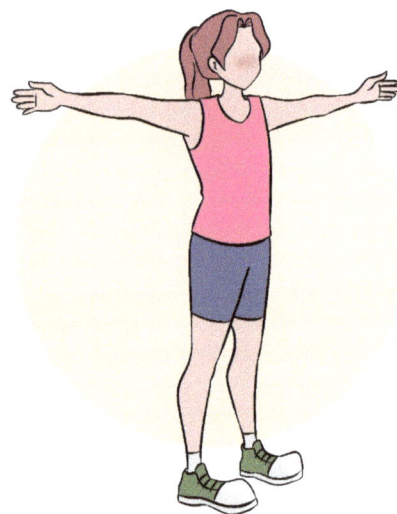

Try It Activities

Start with 10 jumping jacks, followed by 10 high knees, and finish with 10 arm circles. Repeat this warm-up sequence two times.

Cooling Down

After you finish your physical activity, it's time to cool down. Cooling down helps your body relax and recover, preventing muscle soreness. Here are some cool-down exercises to try:

Slow Jog or Walk

After running or playing a sport, slow down your pace and jog or walk slowly for a few minutes. This helps lower your heart rate and returns your body to a resting state.

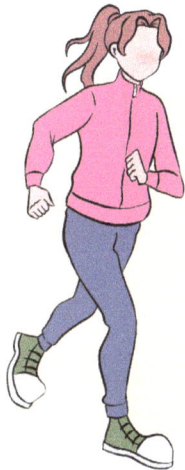

Stretching

Perform gentle stretches for your major muscle groups. Reach for your toes, extend your arms overhead, and do calf stretches. Remember to breathe deeply and hold each stretch for 15-30 seconds.

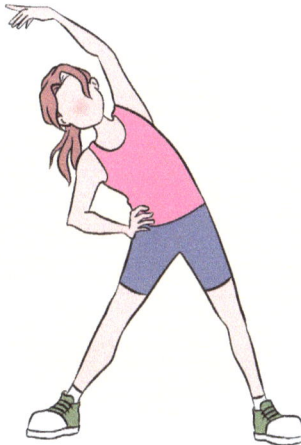

Deep Breathing

Sit or lie down, close your eyes, and take slow, deep breaths. Inhale deeply through your nose, fill your belly with air, and exhale slowly through your mouth. This helps your body relax and promotes a sense of calm.

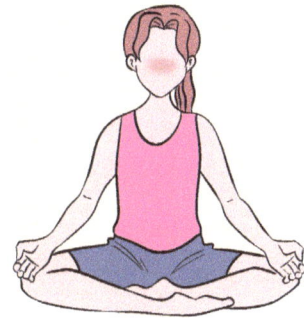

Try It Activities

Cool-Down Exercise: After finishing your physical activity, go for a slow jog or walk for 5 minutes. Then, find a comfortable spot to stretch your legs, arms, and back. Hold each stretch for 15-30 seconds.

Deep Breathing Exercise: Sit or lie down in a quiet place. Close your eyes and take five slow, deep breaths. Inhale through your nose, fill your belly, and exhale through your mouth, letting go of any tension.

Physical Activity

Core Exercises

Supermans

1 Lie face down on the ground with your arms extended in front of you.

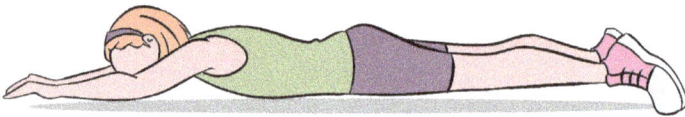

2 Lift your arms, chest, and legs off the ground simultaneously.

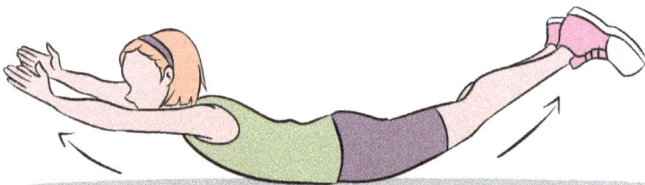

3 Hold this position for a few seconds, squeezing your back and glute muscles.

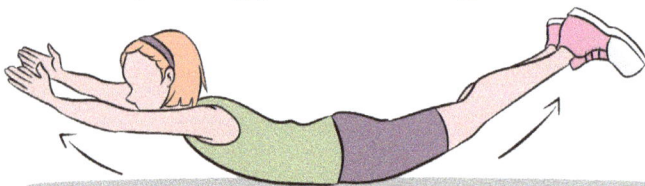

4 Slowly lower your body back down to the starting position.

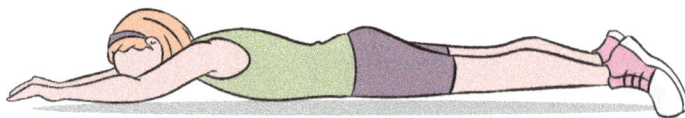

5 Repeat for a set of 6+ repetitions.

Planks

1 Start by lying face down on the floor with your forearms flat on the ground and elbows directly under your shoulders.

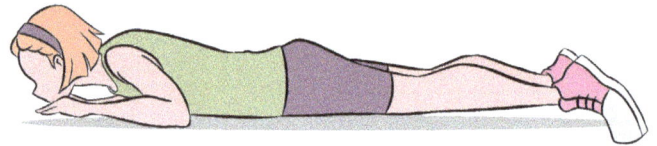

2 Lift your body off the ground, resting on your forearms and toes, keeping your body in a straight line from head to toe.

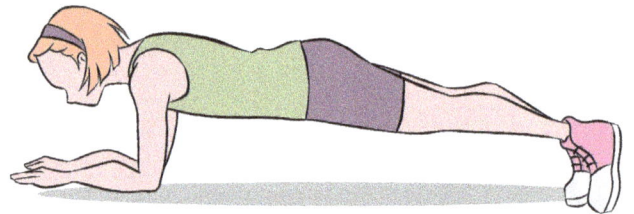

3 Engage your core muscles by squeezing your belly button towards your spine.

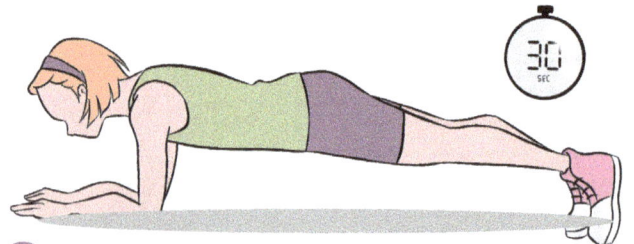

4 Hold the position for 20 to 30 seconds or as long as you can maintain proper form.

Upper Body Exercises

Regular Push-Ups

1 Start in a plank position with your hands slightly wider than shoulder-width apart and aligned with your chest.

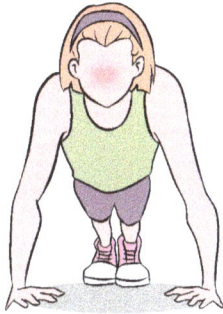

2 Position your feet together or slightly apart, ensuring your body forms a straight line from head to heels.

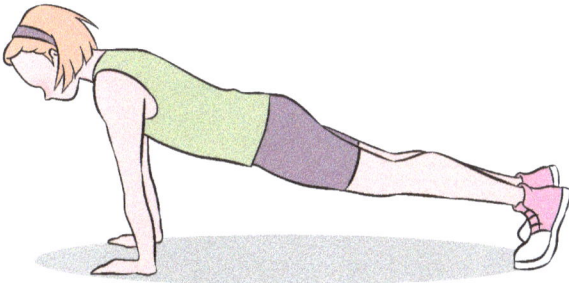

3 Engage your core, glutes, and legs to maintain stability throughout the exercise.

4 Lower your body towards the ground by bending your elbows, keeping them close to your sides.

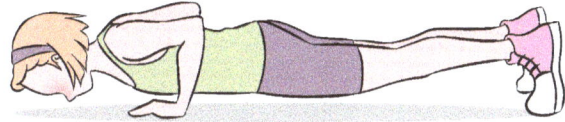

5 Continue descending until your chest is just above the ground or as low as you can comfortably go.

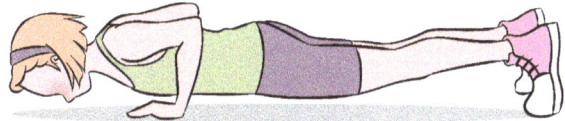

6 Push through your palms, extending your elbows to raise your body back up to the starting position.

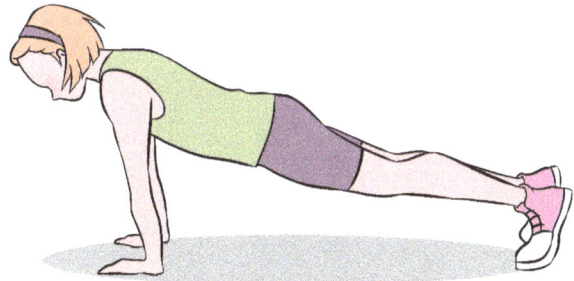

7 Keep your body aligned throughout the movement, avoiding sagging or raising your hips.

8 Repeat for a set of 6+ repetitions.

Wide Push-Ups:

1 Start in a plank position with your hands wider than shoulder-width apart.

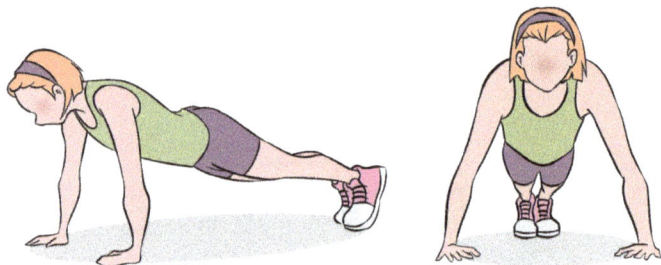

2 Lower your body towards the ground by bending your elbows, keeping your back straight.

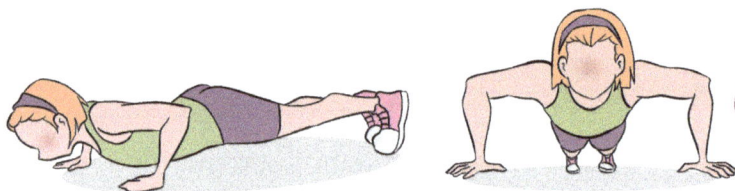

3 Push through your palms to raise your body back up to the starting position.

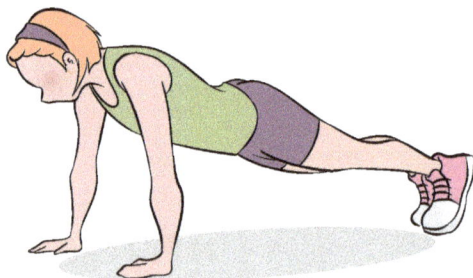

4 Repeat for a set of 6+ repetitions.

Pike Push-Ups:

1 Start in a push-up position with your hands slightly wider than shoulder-width apart and your body forming an inverted V shape. Your hips should be raised, and your heels may be elevated on a step or sturdy surface if desired.

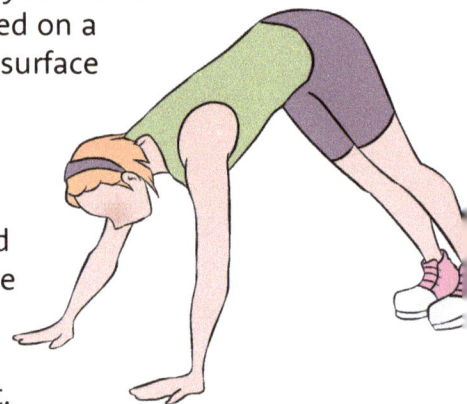

2 Ensure your head is aligned with your spine and your gaze is directed toward your feet.

3 Lower your upper body by bending your elbows, allowing your head to move between your arms as you descend.

4 Keep your core engaged and maintain control as you push back up to the starting position, fully extending

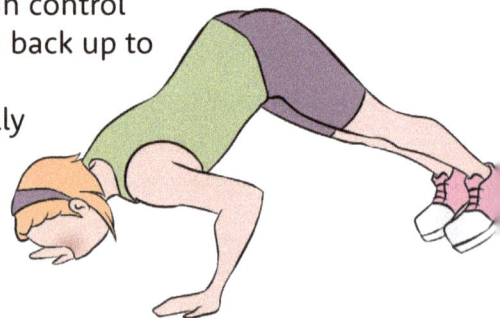

5 Repeat for a set of 6+ repetitions.

Tips for proper push-up form:

1 Maintain a neutral spine by looking slightly ahead, not upward or downward.

2 Keep your elbows close to your sides, which helps engage the triceps and shoulders.

3 Breathe naturally throughout the exercise, exhaling as you push up and inhaling as you lower down.

4 If the full push-up is challenging, you can modify it by performing them on your knees instead of your toes.

5 Regular push-ups are an effective compound exercise that strengthens multiple muscle groups, including the shoulders. As with any exercise, listening to your body, starting at a comfortable level, and gradually increasing intensity as you build strength is essential.

Traditional Pull-Ups:

1 Find a pull-up bar or sturdy horizontal structure that can support your weight.

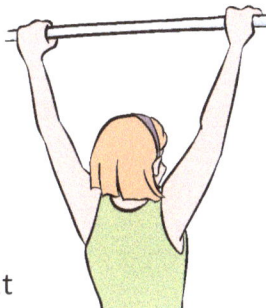

2 Grasp the bar with an overhand grip, slightly wider than shoulder-width apart.

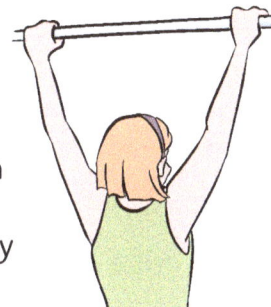

3 Hang with your arms fully extended and your feet off the ground.

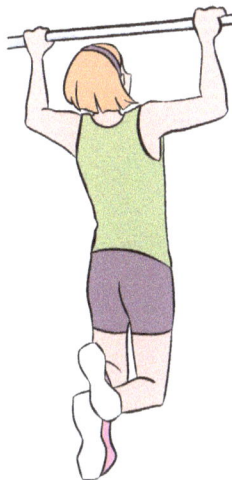

4 Engage your core and pull yourself up by bending your elbows and lifting your body until your chin clears the bar.

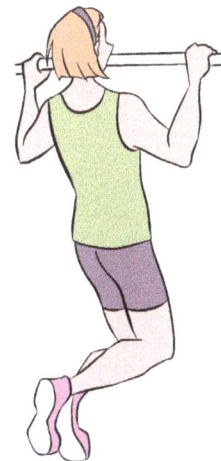

5 Lower your body back down with control until your arms are fully extended.

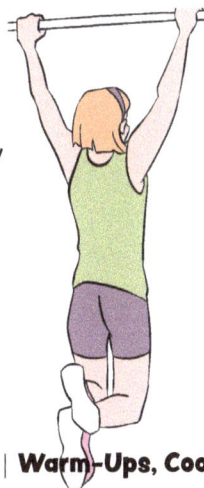

6 Repeat for a set of 6+ repetitions.

Pull-Ups Progressions (If not ready for a full traditional pull-up):

A full pull-up can be challenging, but it's attainable with a well-structured progression plan and consistent effort. Here's a step-by-step plan to help you progress toward a full pull-up:

1 **Build overall upper body strength:** Start by focusing on different Push-ups.

2 **Negatives:** Stand on an elevated surface or use a chair to start in the top position of the pull-up, with your chin above the bar. Slowly lower yourself down, taking around 3-5 seconds to descend. Repeat as many times as you can.

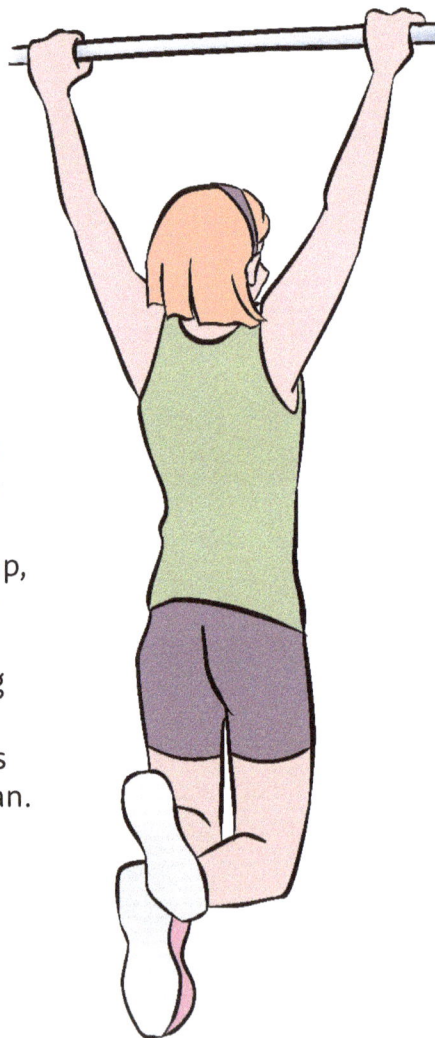

3 **Isometric holds:** Start with your arms at the bottom position and hold for as long as possible. Gradually work towards holding at different angles until you can hold at the halfway point and then close to the top.

4 **Full pull-up progression:** Once you have developed sufficient strength and can easily perform the earlier progressions, attempt a full pull-up. Start with a partial range of motion and gradually work towards a full pull-up by increasing your range over time.

Lower Body Exercises

Regular Squats:

1. Stand with your feet shoulder-width apart, toes pointing slightly outward.

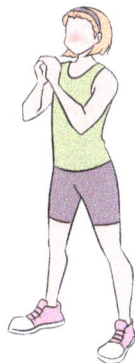

2. Bend your knees and push your hips back like sitting in a chair.

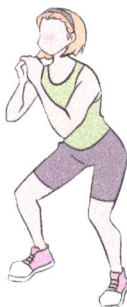

3. Keep your chest lifted and your weight on your heels.

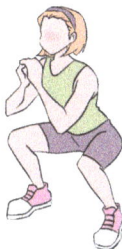

4. Lower your body until your thighs are parallel to the ground.

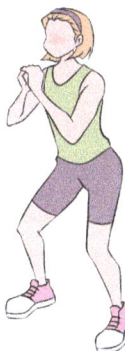

5. Push through your heels to return to the starting position.

6. Repeat for a set of 6+ repetitions.

Sumo Squats:

1. Stand with your feet wider than shoulder-width apart, and toes pointed slightly outward.

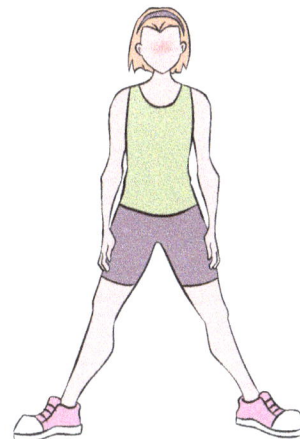

2. Lower your body into a squat, keeping your knees aligned with your toes and your chest lifted.

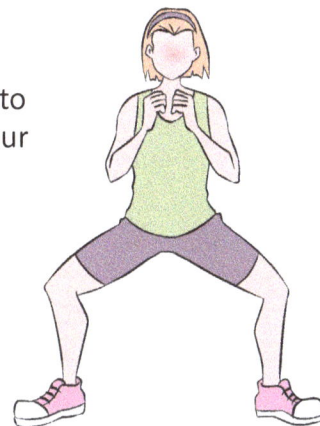

3. Push through your heels to raise your body back up to the starting position.

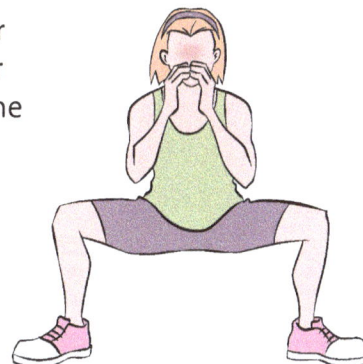

4. Repeat for a set of 6+ repetitions.

Frog Jumps:

1 Start in a squat position with your feet shoulder-width apart and your hands on the ground in front of you.

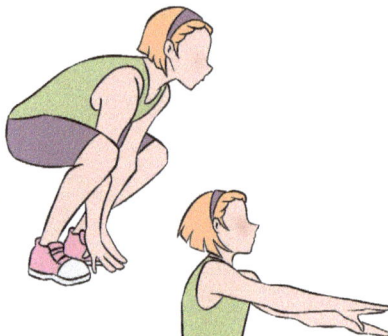

2 Jump forward as far as possible, landing in a squat position.

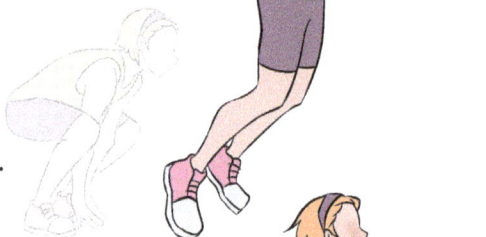

3 Swing your arms forward for momentum.

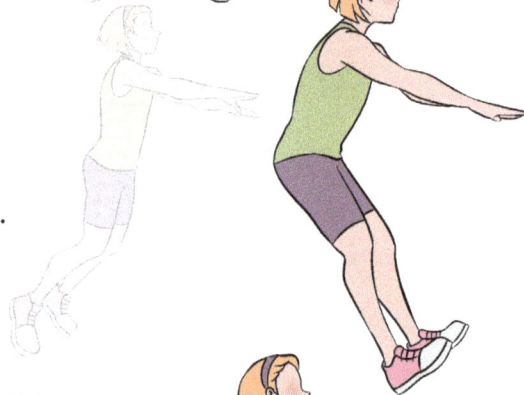

4 Jump again, this time jumping backward to your starting position.

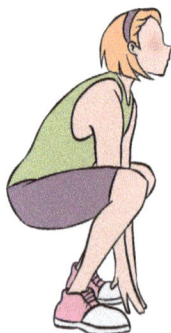

5 Repeat for a set of 6+ repetitions.

Forward Lunges:

1 Stand tall with your feet hip-width apart.

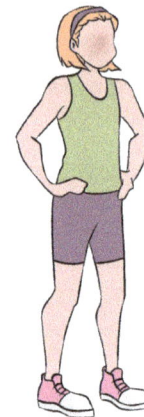

2 Take a big step forward with your right foot, lowering your body until your right knee is at a 90-degree angle.

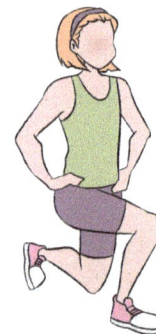

3 Push through your right heel to return to the starting position.

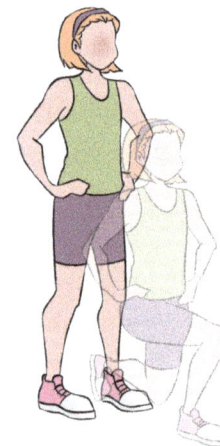

4 Repeat with your left leg.

5 Alternate legs and do a set of 6+ repetitions on each side.

Reverse Lunges:

1. Stand tall with your feet hip-width apart.

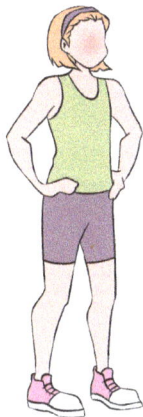

2. Take a big step backward with your left foot, lowering your body until your left knee is at a 90-degree angle.

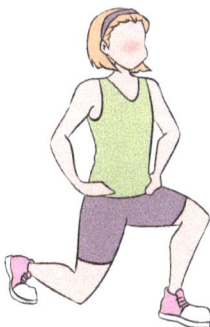

3. Push through your left heel to return to the starting position.

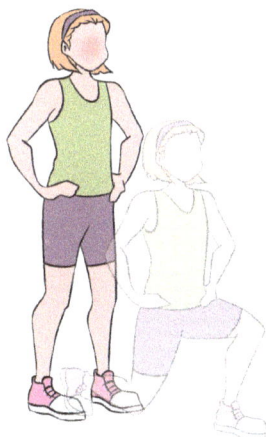

4. Repeat with your right leg.

5. Alternate legs and do a set of 6+ repetitions on each side.

Side Lunges:

1. Stand with your feet wider than shoulder-width apart, toes pointing forward.

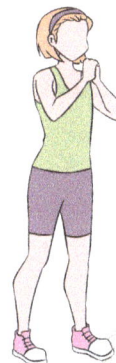

2. Shift your body weight to the right side, bending your right knee and keeping your left leg straight.

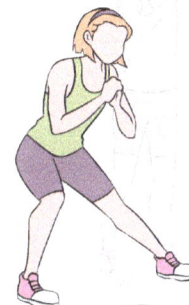

3. Push through your right heel to return to the starting position.

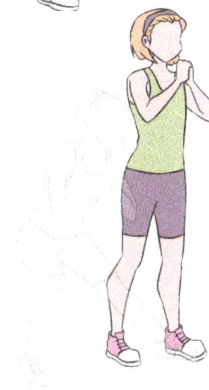

4. Repeat on the left side.

5. Alternate sides and do a set of 6+ repetitions on each side.

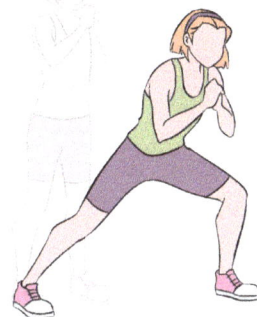

Once you get the hang of the basics, here is a three-day per week, whole body, bodyweight program to try out. Most importantly, before you begin any workout routine, check with your parents and doctor to ensure you can do all the in this program as detailed on the previous pages.

Workout 1:
Monday

Excercise	Sets x Reps
Planks	3 x 20-30 sec
Regular Squats	3 x 6+
Regular Push-Ups	3 x 6+
Sumo Squats	3 x 6+
Wide Push-Ups	3 x 6+

Workout 2:
Wednesday

Excercise	Sets x Reps
Supermans	3 x 6+
Lunges (Forward and Reverse)	3 x 6+ (each side)
Regular Push-Ups	3 x 6+
Side Lunges	3 x 6+ (each side)
Traditional or Assisted Pull-Ups	3 x 6+

Workout 3:
Friday

Excercise	Sets x Reps
Planks	3 x 20-30 sec
Frog Jumps	3 x 6+
Regular Push-Ups	3 x 6+
Regular Squats	3 x 6+
Pike Push-Ups	3 x 6+

"

Remember, finding enjoyable activities is key to a healthy and active lifestyle. Warm-up and cool down properly to keep your body happy and strong. So, get out there and have fun.

Chapter 4

Martial Arts
and Mobility

Get ready to discover the world of martial arts and unlock your full potential. Martial arts are not just about cool moves and fancy kicks; they also help build confidence, flexibility, coordination, and balance.

The Power of Martial Arts

Martial arts are more than self-defense techniques. They are ancient practices that teach discipline, respect, and self-control while helping you stay fit and agile. Martial arts boost your physical abilities and strengthen your mind and spirit. So, let's discover some popular martial arts styles and their benefits!

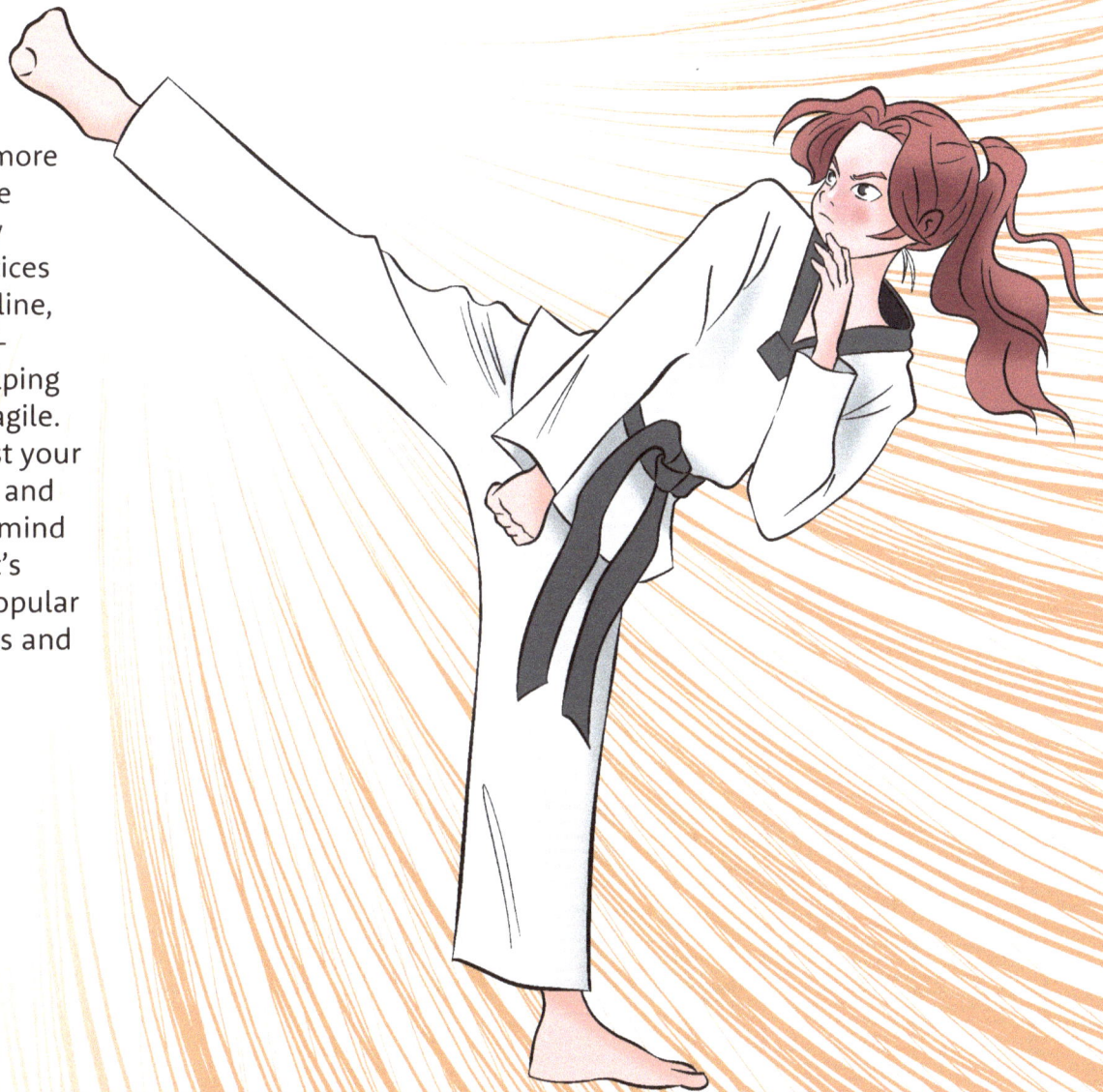

Taekwondo:
Taekwondo combines fast kicks, punches, and powerful movements. It improves your balance, agility, and self-confidence.

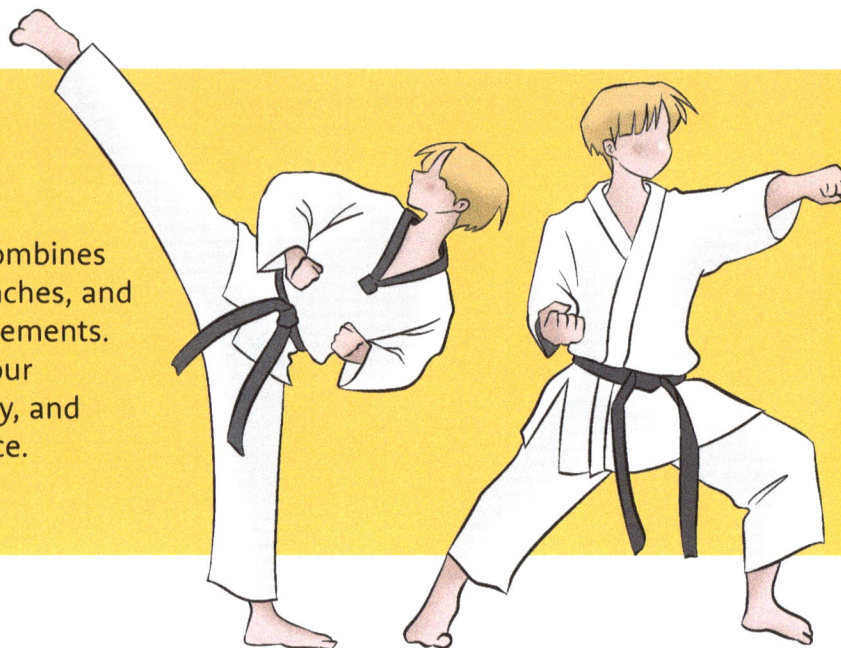

Karate:
Karate focuses on strikes, kicks, and blocking techniques. It enhances your strength, speed, and discipline.

Aikido:
Aikido emphasizes using an opponent's energy to defend yourself. It enhances your flexibility, balance, and harmony of movement.

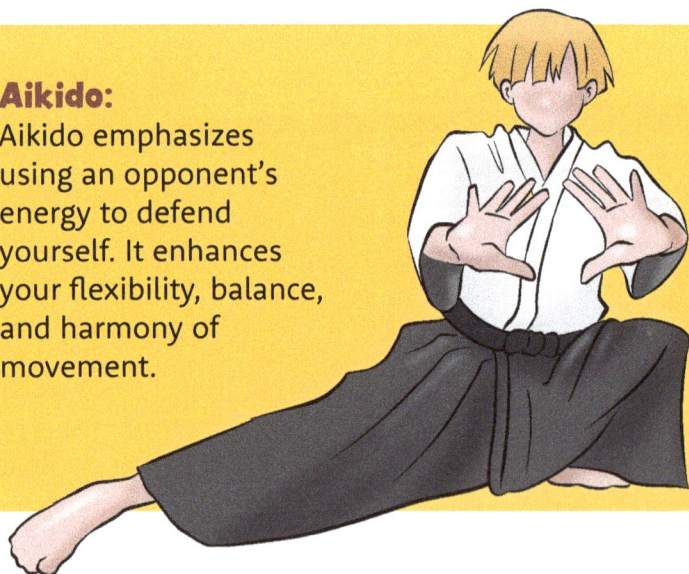

Jiu-Jitsu:
Jiu-jitsu teaches ground fighting and submission holds. It improves your grappling skills, body awareness, and problem-solving abilities.

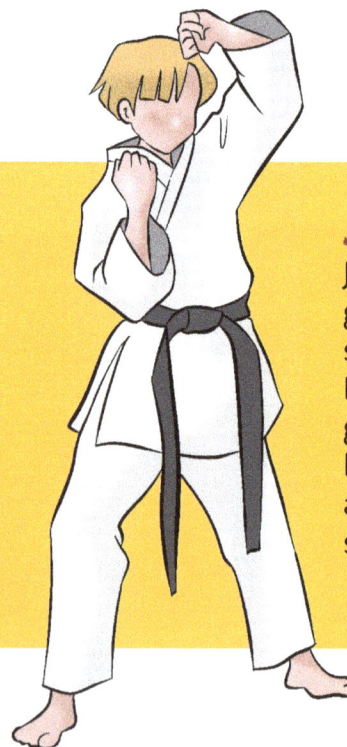

Krav Maga:
Krav Maga is a practical self-defense system. It enhances your overall fitness, situational awareness, and self-defense skills.

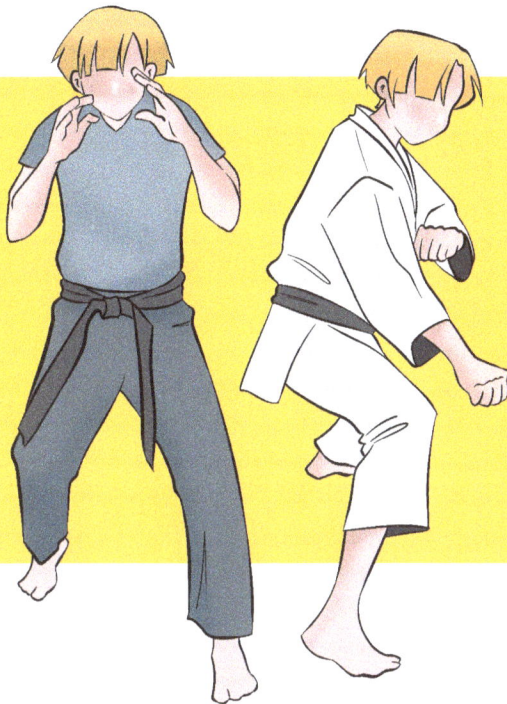

Judo:
Judo focuses on throws, holds, and ground techniques. It develops your strength, coordination, and mental resilience.

Boxing:
Boxing involves punches, footwork, and defensive techniques. It enhances your speed, hand-eye coordination, and cardiovascular fitness.

Jeet Kune Do:
Jeet Kune Do combines various martial arts techniques. It promotes adaptability, creativity, and fluidity of movement.

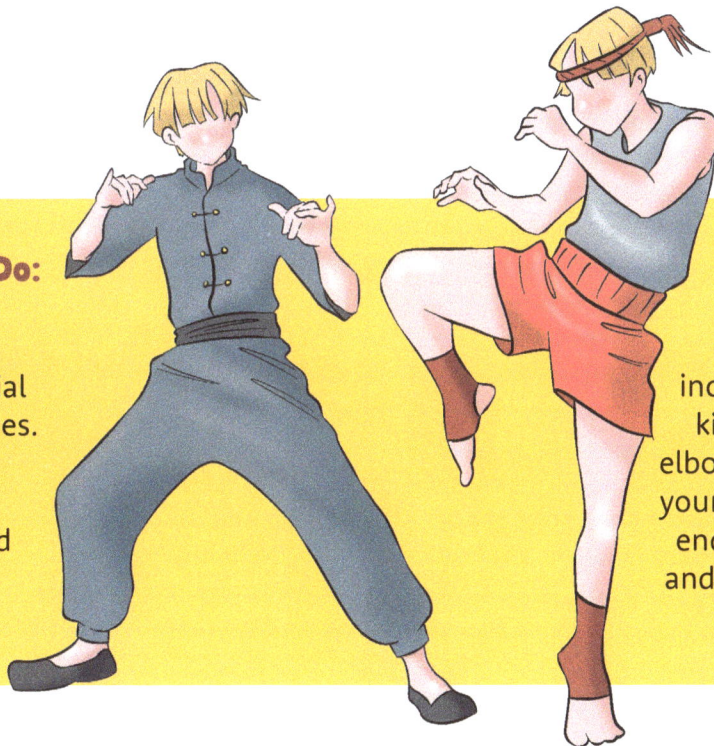

Muay Thai:
Muay Thai is a martial art that includes punches, kicks, knees, and elbows. It improves your cardiovascular endurance, agility, and striking power.

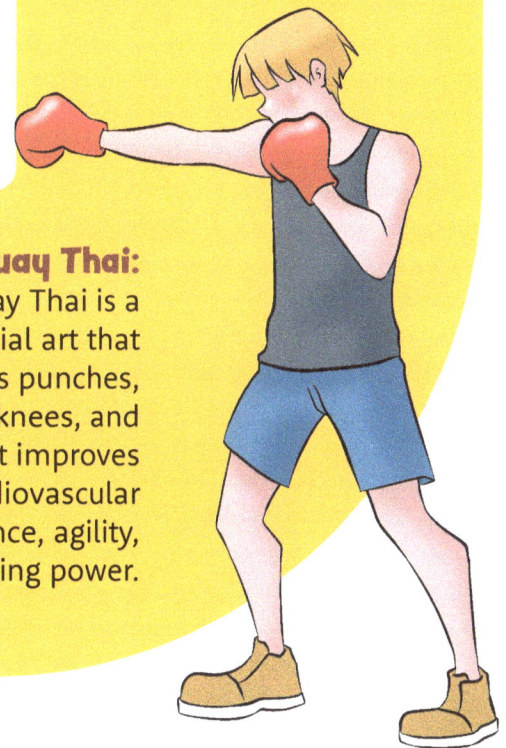

Try It Activities

1. Basic Punches and Kicks:

Stand with your feet shoulder-width apart. Practice throwing punches (jab, cross, hook) and kicks (front kick, roundhouse kick) in the air. Start slowly and gradually increase your speed and power.

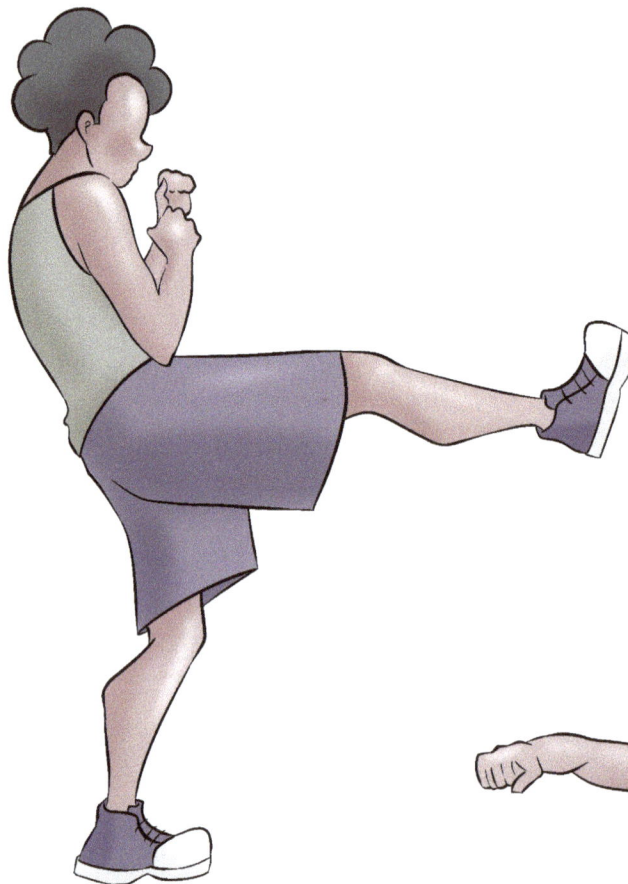

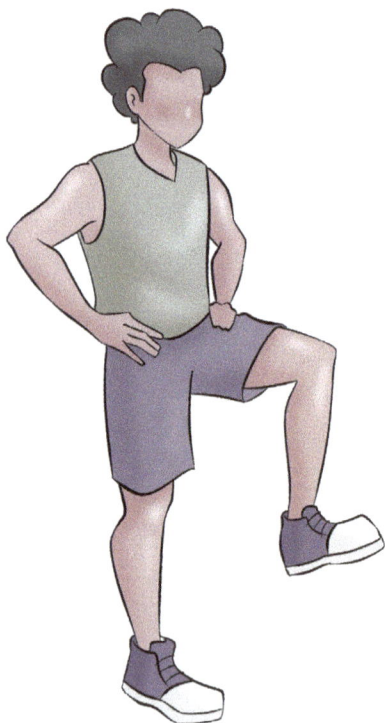

2. Balance Exercises:

Stand on one leg and hold your balance for as long as possible. Switch legs and repeat. You can also try standing on one leg while kicking forward or sideways.

3. Shadow Sparring:

Pretend you're sparring with an imaginary opponent. Practice your punches, kicks, and footwork, moving around and dodging imaginary attacks. Stay light on your feet and focus on your form and technique.

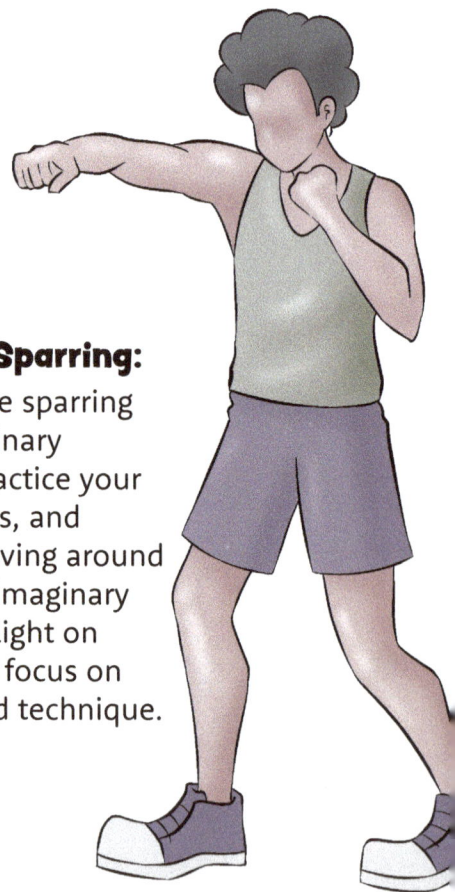

Remember, martial arts require discipline and practice. Find a reputable martial arts school or instructor to learn the techniques safely. Always warm up before training and listen to your body to avoid injuries. Martial arts will improve physical fitness and boost confidence and mental focus. So, embrace the warrior's way and unleash your inner martial artist!

Chapter 5

Hydration, Electrolytes, And Limiting Sugary Drinks

In this chapter, we'll dive into hydration, electrolytes, and why limiting sugary drinks like soda or energy drinks is important. So grab your water bottles, and let's start on this exciting journey to quench your thirst healthily!

The Power of Hydration

Did you know that water is like magic fuel for your body? It keeps you energized, helps your organs work correctly, and keeps your skin glowing. Staying hydrated means drinking enough water to keep your body in tip-top shape. It's super important, especially during physical activities and hot weather, when your body sweats more and needs extra hydration. So, let's explore why hydration is crucial and how to make it a part of your daily routine!

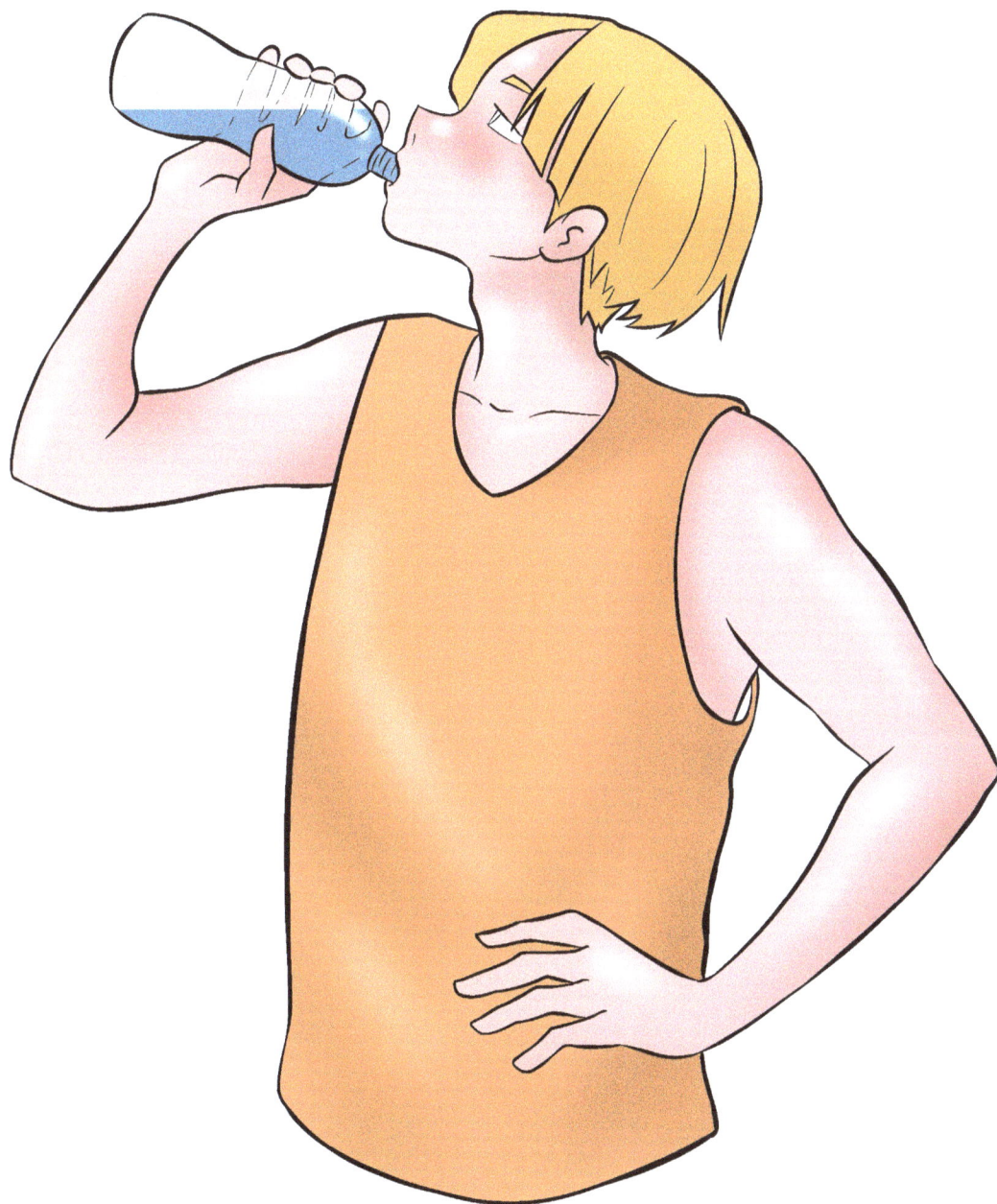

Electrolytes:
The Mighty Minerals

Now, let's meet some incredible minerals called electrolytes! These unique minerals, like sodium, potassium, calcium, and magnesium, are like little messengers in your body. They help your cells talk to each other, maintain the right balance of fluids, and support essential functions like muscle contractions and nerve impulses. Electrolytes are your body's sidekicks in the hydration game!

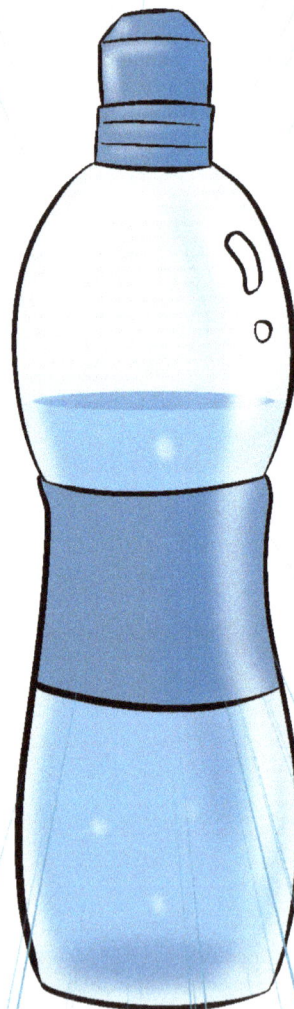

Tips for Staying Hydrated

Drink Plenty of Water: Carry a water bottle with you wherever you go and take sips throughout the day. Drink when you are thirsty, and if you have access to them and parental approval, try out electrolyte powders. Electrolyte powders are a convenient option to enhance the mineral content of your water. These powders usually contain sodium, potassium, calcium, and magnesium.

Hydrate During Physical Activities: When playing sports, dancing, or having fun outdoors, drink water before, during, and after your activities to replenish the fluids you lose through sweat.

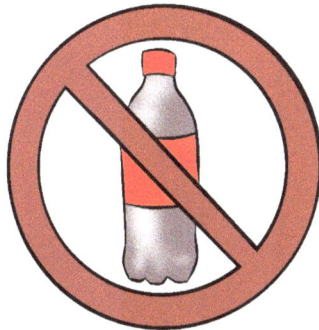

Limit Sugary Drinks: While sugary drinks seem tempting, they can be sneaky villains that harm your health. They often have too much added sugar, harming your teeth and overall well-being. So, limit soda, energy drinks, and other sugary beverages.

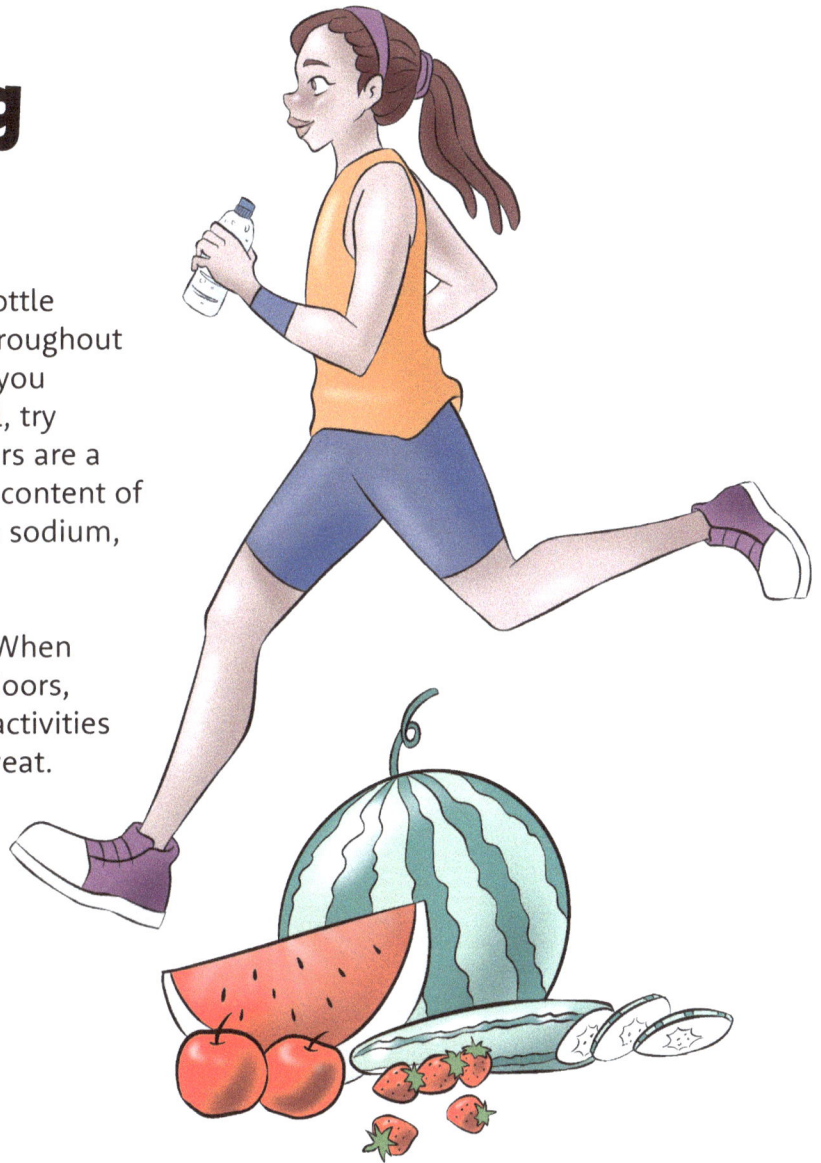

Eat Hydrating Foods: Enjoy delicious fruits and vegetables like watermelon, oranges, cucumbers, and strawberries that have high water content. They not only taste yummy but also help keep you hydrated.

Try It Activities

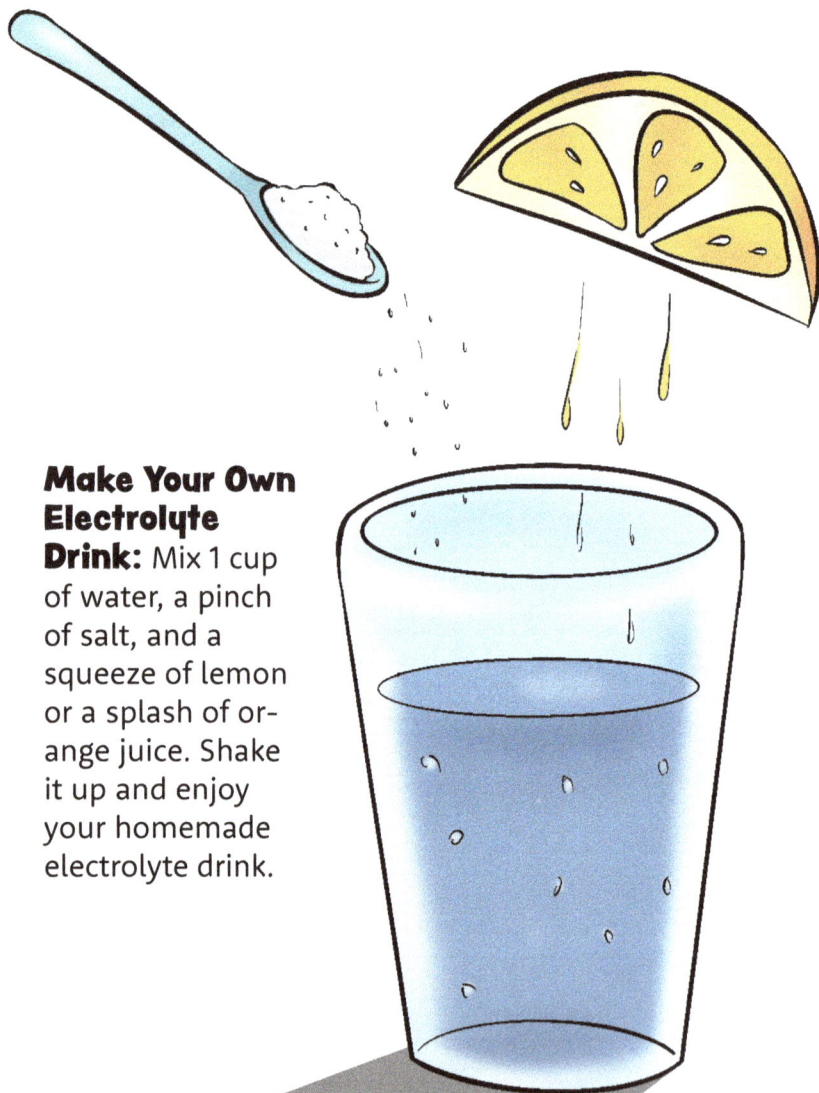

Hydration Tracker: Create a fun chart or use stickers to track how many glasses of water you drink each day. Aim to reach your 6-8 glasses goal and celebrate each milestone!

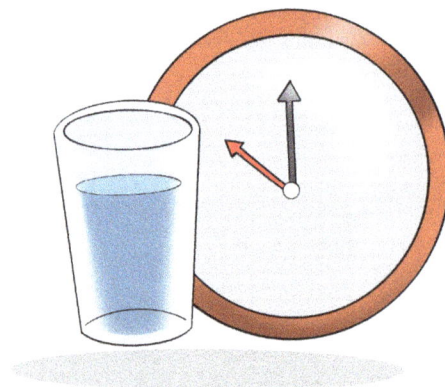

Make Your Own Electrolyte Drink: Mix 1 cup of water, a pinch of salt, and a squeeze of lemon or a splash of orange juice. Shake it up and enjoy your homemade electrolyte drink.

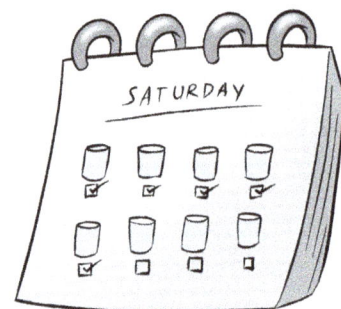

Hydration Breaks: Set a timer on your watch or ask an adult to remind you to take hydration breaks every hour. Get up, stretch, and sip water to keep your body hydrated throughout the day.

"

Remember, staying hydrated helps you feel your best all of the time. Drink water, enjoy hydrating foods, and limit sugary drinks to keep your body happy and healthy. So, raise your water bottles and toast to hydration's excellent benefits! Cheers to a hydrated you!

Chapter 6

Balanced Diet, Mindful Eating, and Portion Control

This chapter will dive into balanced diets, mindful eating, and portion control. Let's get started!

Balanced Diet

Your body needs different nutrients to grow, stay healthy, and keep active. Here are some superstars that should be on your plate:

Fruits: These colorful and juicy wonders are packed with vitamins and minerals. Think apples, oranges, berries, and bananas. They make great snacks or additions to your meals.

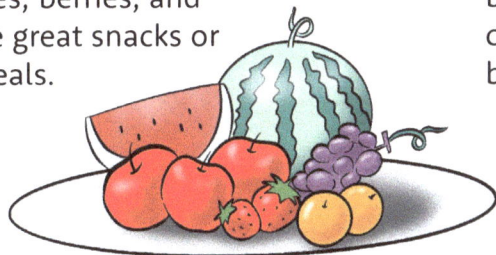

Healthy Fats: Not all fats are bad! Some fats are essential for your body. Avocados, nuts, and olive oil contain healthy fats that keep your brain and heart happy.

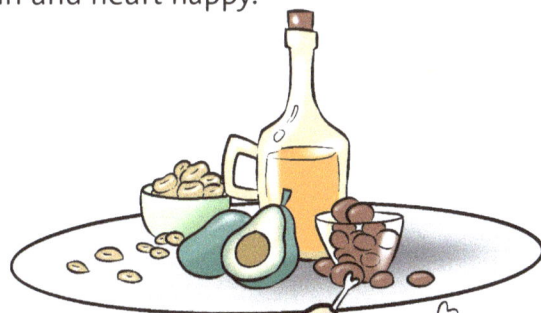

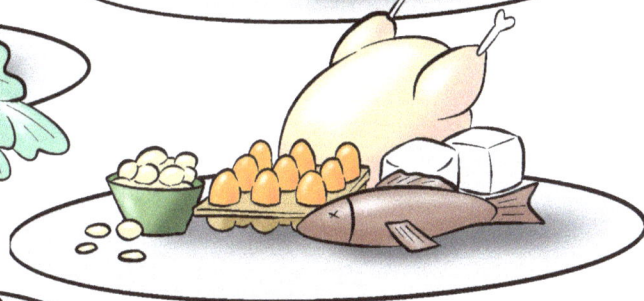

Veggies:
Green, red, orange, and yellow vegetables are like nature's superheroes. They are rich in fiber, vitamins, and minerals. Fill your plate with broccoli, carrots, spinach, and bell peppers.

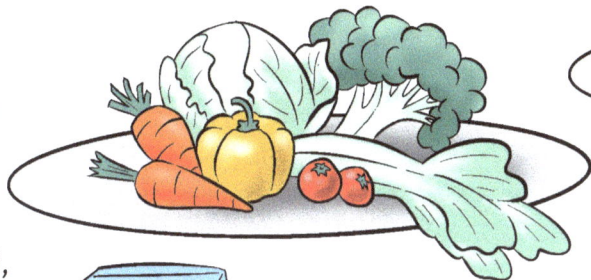

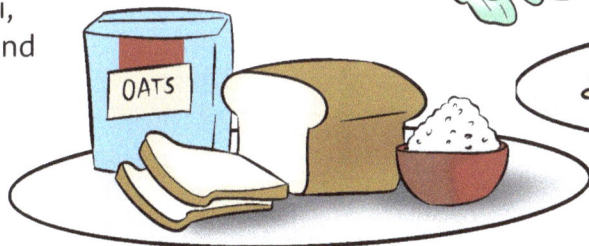

Whole Grains: Whole wheat bread, brown rice, and oats haven't lost their nutritious parts during processing. They provide you with energy and essential nutrients like fiber.

Proteins: Proteins are building blocks for your body. They help repair and grow your muscles and keep you strong. Look for sources like beef, chicken, fish, beans, tofu, and eggs.

Mindful Eating

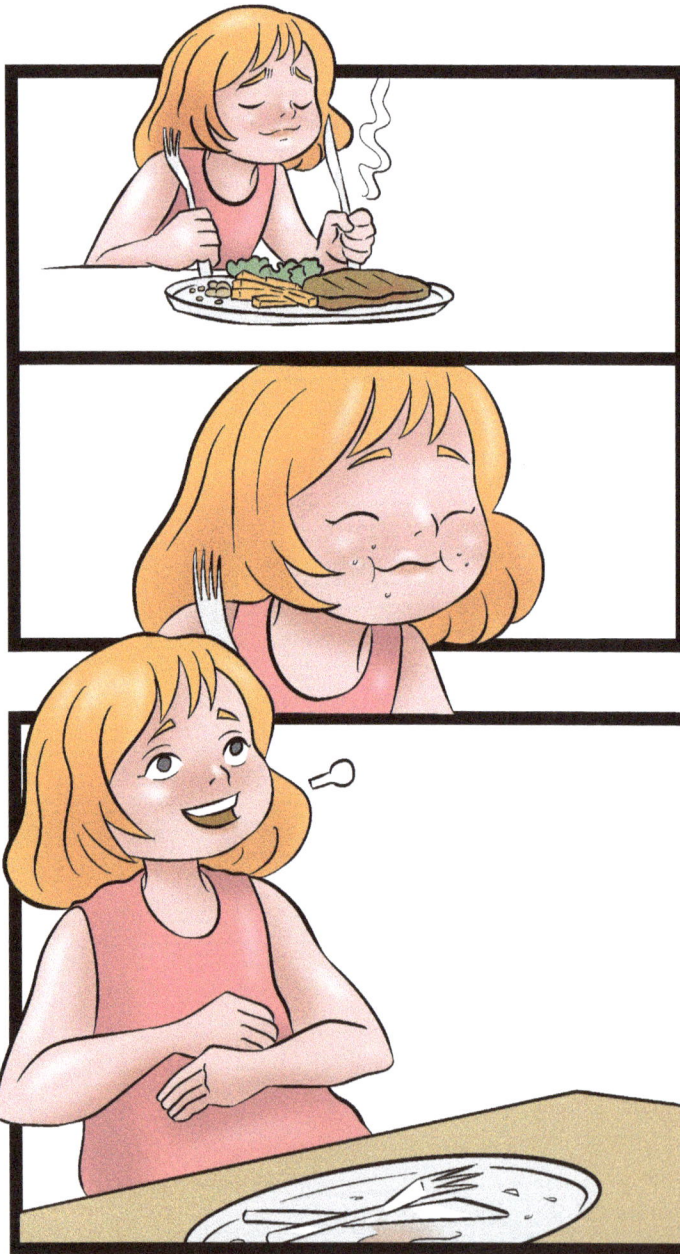

Have you ever rushed through a meal without enjoying it? Mindful eating is all about slowing down and savoring your food. Here's how you can practice it:

Pay attention:
Sit at the table and focus on your meal. Notice the colors, smells, and flavors of the food.

Chew well:
Take small bites and chew your food slowly. This helps your body digest food properly and maximize nutrient absorption.

Listen to your body:
Pay attention to your hunger and fullness cues. Eat when you're hungry and stop when you're comfortably satisfied. Your body knows best!

Portion Control

Portion control means eating the right amount of food for your body. Here are some tips to help

Use smaller plates and bowls: It tricks your mind into thinking you're eating more.

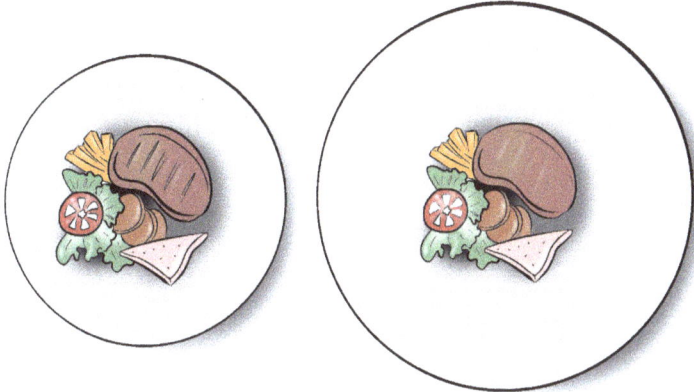

Serve yourself just enough: Start with small portions and have more if you're still hungry.

Eat slowly: Give your body time to register when it's full.

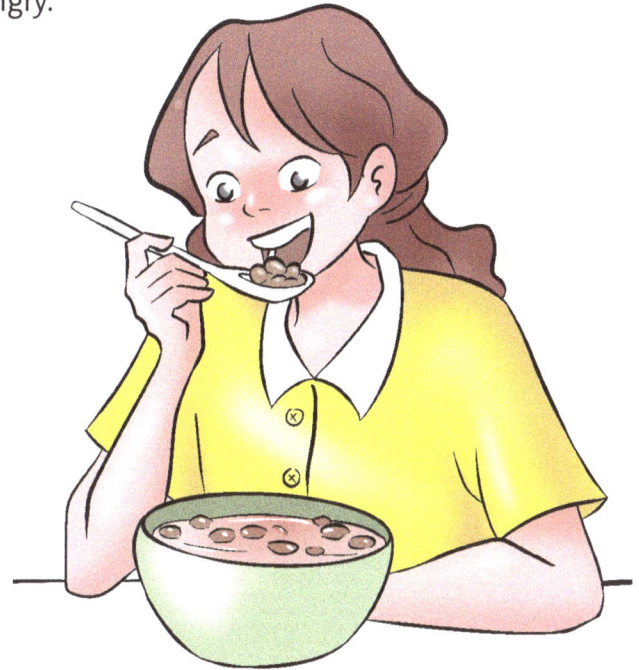

Enjoy treats in moderation: It's okay to have your favorite snacks or desserts, but remember to keep them in balance with the rest of your meals.

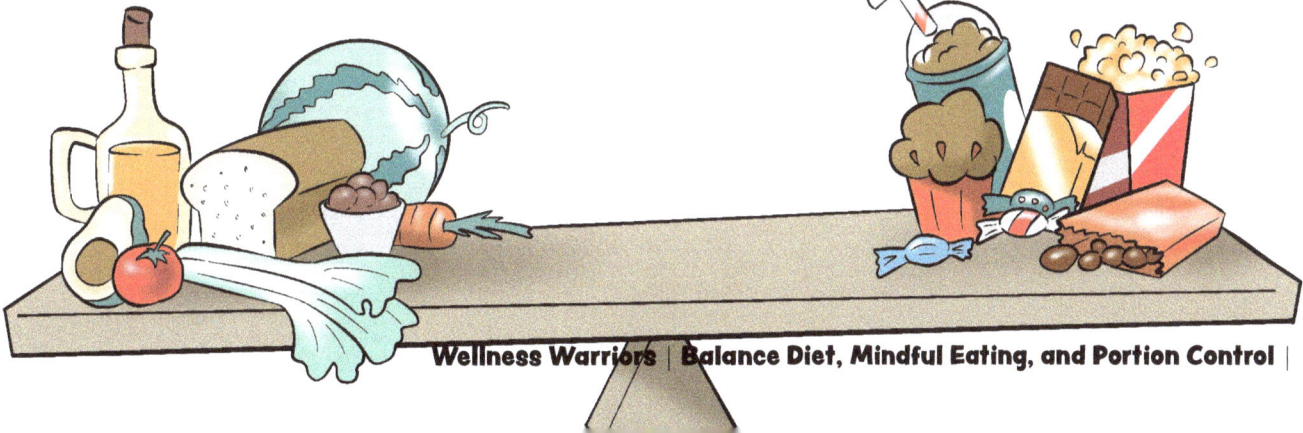

Try It Activities

Create a colorful meal: Draw a picture or describe a balanced meal with fruits, veggies, whole grains, proteins, and healthy fats.

Mindful eating challenge: Pick one meal or snack daily to practice mindful eating. Sit at the table, focus on your food, and eat slowly, paying attention to the flavors and textures.

Portion control game: Use different-sized bowls or plates and practice serving yourself appropriate portion sizes for different types of food. See if you can get it just right!

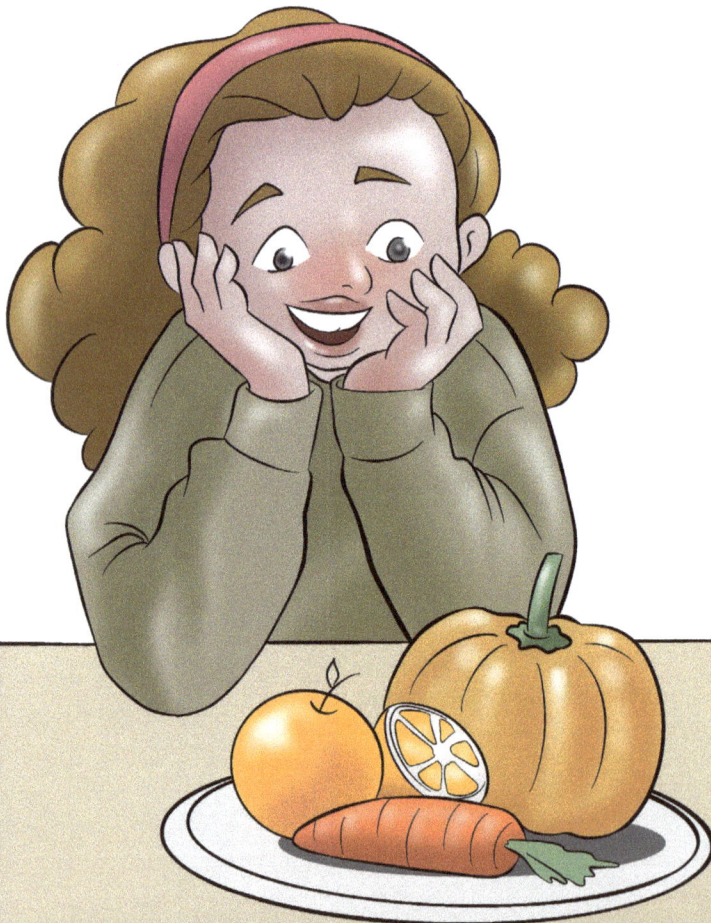

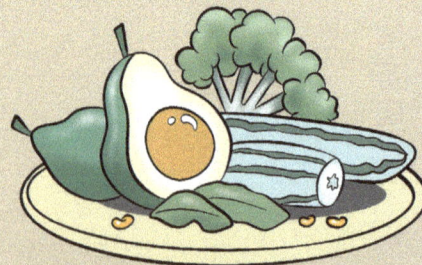

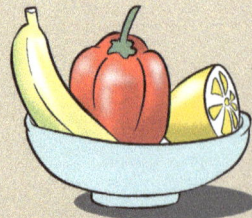

"

Remember, a balanced diet, mindful eating, and portion control are all about taking care of your body and healthily enjoying food. Keep exploring and discovering new tasty and nutritious foods. Bon appétit!

Chapter 7

Healthy Snacking,
Cooking, and Meal Preparation

Hey there, little chefs! Get your aprons ready because we're about to dive into the beautiful world of healthy snacking, cooking, and meal preparation. Make sure you first talk with your parents or guardians before you do any cooking or even preparation for cooking.

Healthy Snacking

Snacks can be both tasty and nutritious. Here are some ideas for delicious and healthy snacks:

Fruity Delight:
Slice fresh fruits like apples, oranges, or berries. They make a refreshing and sweet snack.

Crunchy Veggies:
Carrot sticks, cucumber slices, and bell pepper strips are perfect for dipping into hummus or yogurt.

Trail Mix Magic:
Mix a handful of nuts, dried fruits, and a sprinkle of whole grain cereal for a crunchy and energizing snack.

Cooking Adventures

Cooking is not only fun, but it also allows you to create delicious meals from scratch. Here are a few cooking methods you can explore:

Baking: Try baking your own healthy muffins, cookies, or even homemade pizza. It's like magic watching them rise in the oven!

Grilling: Fire up the grill and cook some tasty vegetables, chicken skewers, or fish. Grilled food has a unique smoky flavor.

Steaming: Steaming vegetables help retain their nutrients and vibrant colors. It's a simple and healthy way to cook broccoli, carrots, or green beans.

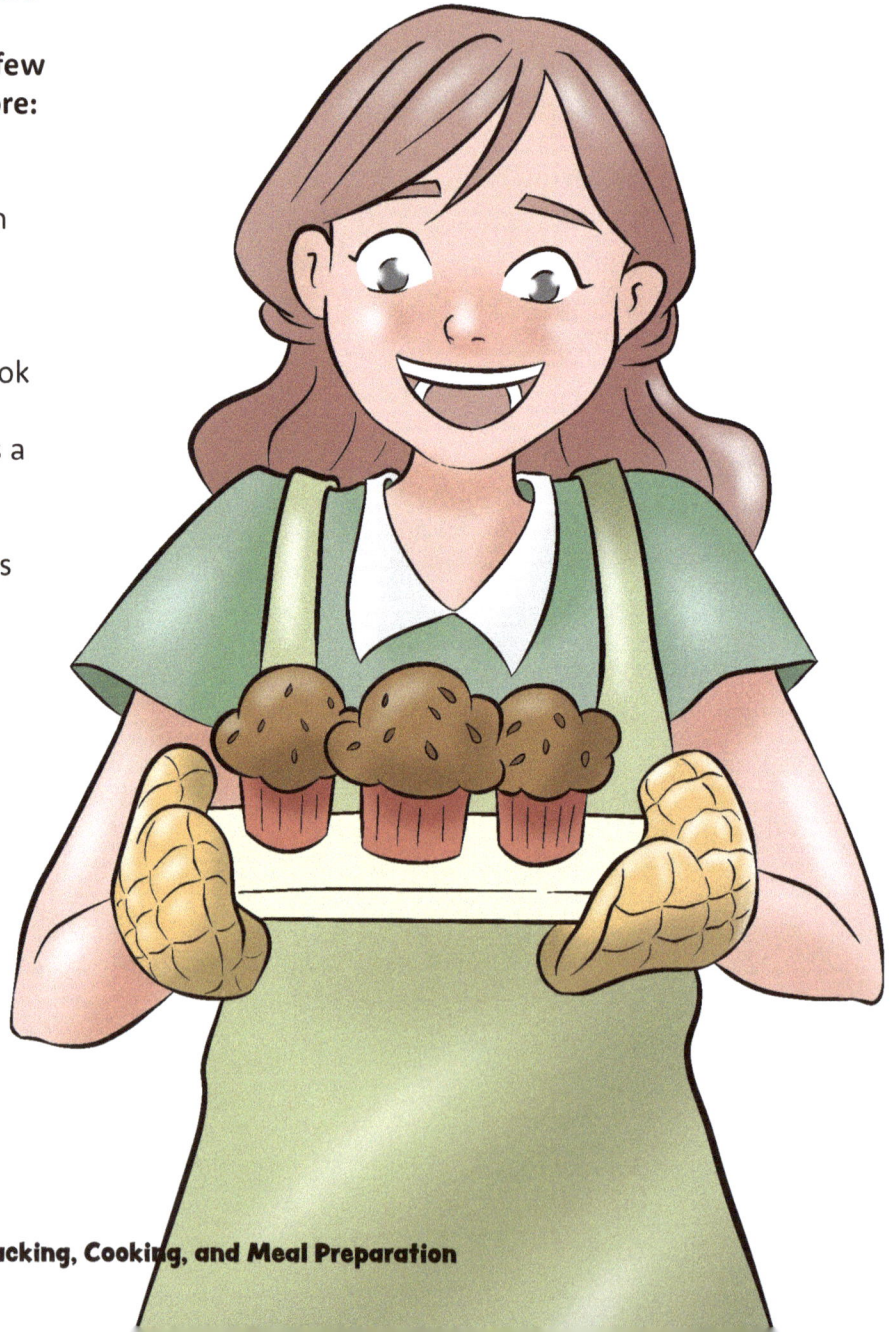

Meal Preparation

Meal preparation is like being your own personal chef. It involves planning and preparing meals in advance, which can save time and make healthy eating easier. Here are some tips to get started:

Plan your meals: Sit down with your family and decide what meals you'll have for the week. Include a variety of fruits, veggies, whole grains, and proteins.

Make a shopping list: Write down all the ingredients you need for your planned meals. It will help you stay organized at the grocery store.

Prep ahead: Spend time washing, cutting, and portioning fruits and vegetables. You can store them in containers for easy access during the week.

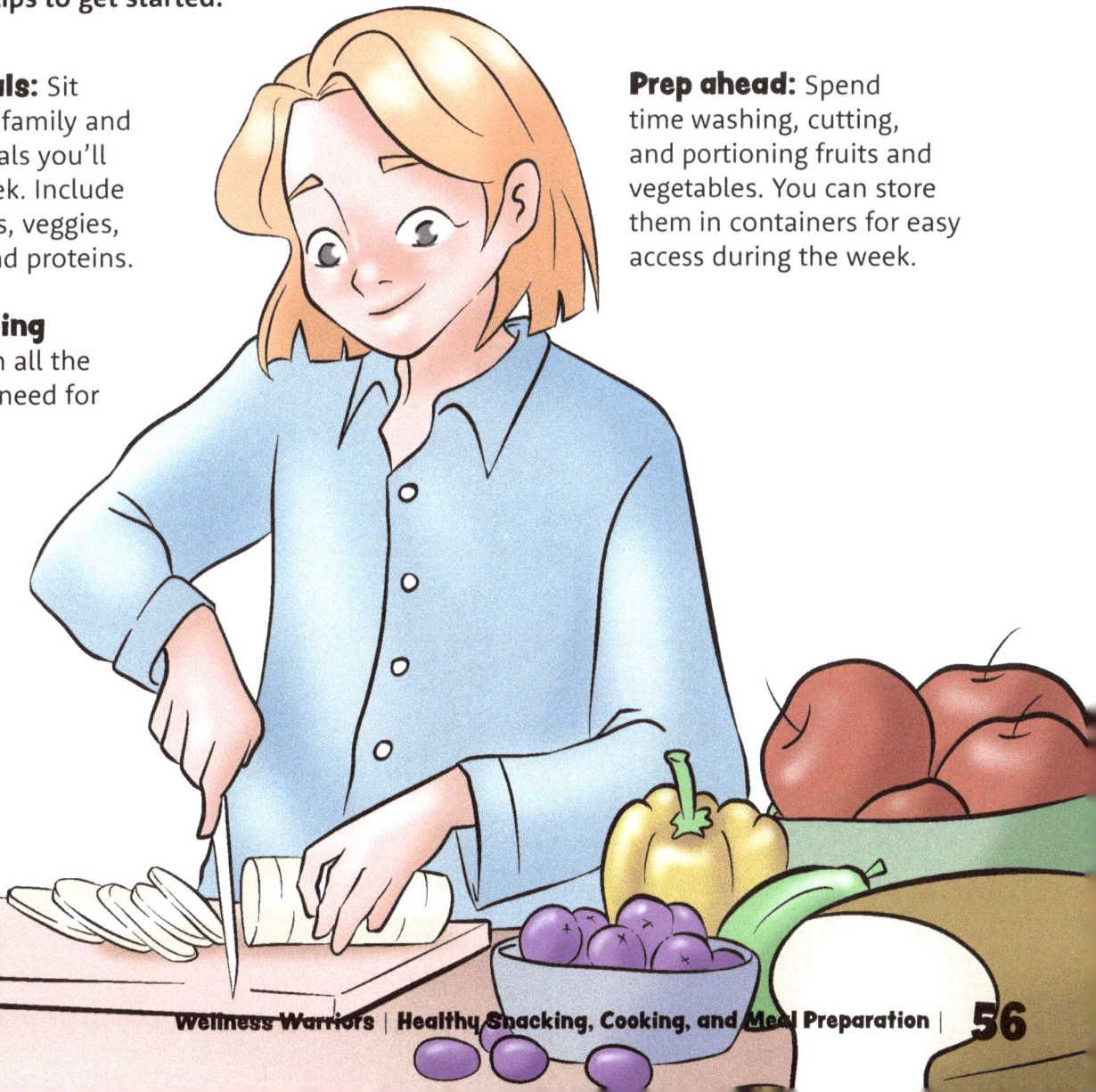

Try It Activities

Create your own snack mix: Mix nuts, dried fruits, and a small amount of dark chocolate or whole-grain cereal. Write down your recipe and share it with your friends.

Cooking challenge: With the help of an adult, choose a simple recipe and prepare it together. It could be a salad, a pasta dish, or a healthy dessert. Enjoy the fruits of your labor!

Meal planning game: Sit with your family and plan a healthy meal for each day of the week. Write down the ingredients you'll need and help create a shopping list.

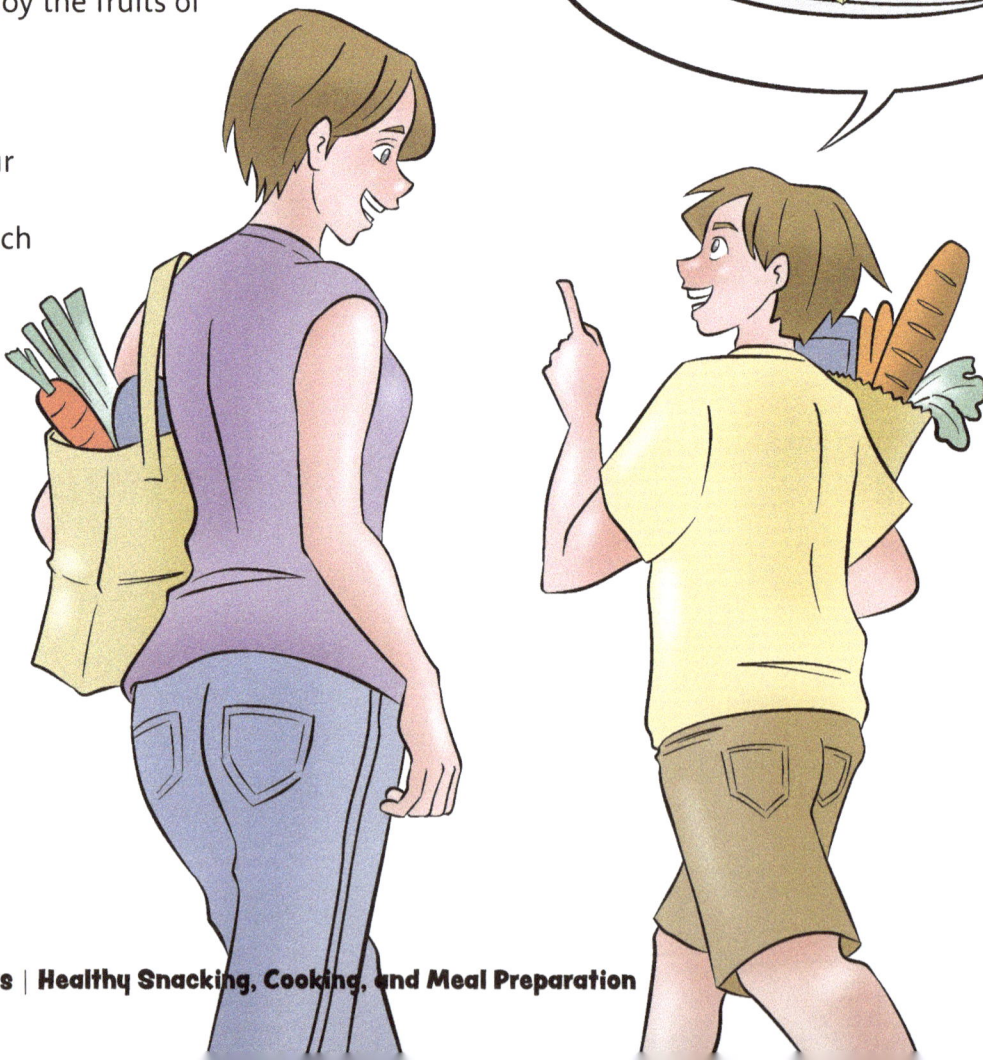

"

Remember, cooking and meal preparation is not only about making tasty food but also about making healthy choices. Get creative, try new ingredients, and have fun in the kitchen. Enjoy the satisfaction of preparing meals that nourish your body and bring joy to your taste buds.

Chapter 8
Dental Health

Get ready to learn all about dental health and how to keep your pearly whites shining bright. Caring for your teeth is essential for a healthy mouth and overall well-being. Make never getting a cavity a top life goal. This will further help you think about taking care of your teeth each day. Are you ready to show off that beautiful smile? Let's dive in!

Brushing Basics

Brushing your teeth is the foundation of good dental hygiene. Here's what you need to know:

Brush at least twice daily: Use a soft-bristled toothbrush and either fluoride or fluoride free toothpaste, as recommended by your dentist. Brush in gentle, circular motions for about two minutes.

Reach all areas: Remember to brush your teeth' front, back, and chewing surfaces. Take your time and be thorough.

Clean your tongue: Gently brush your tongue to remove bacteria and keep your breath.

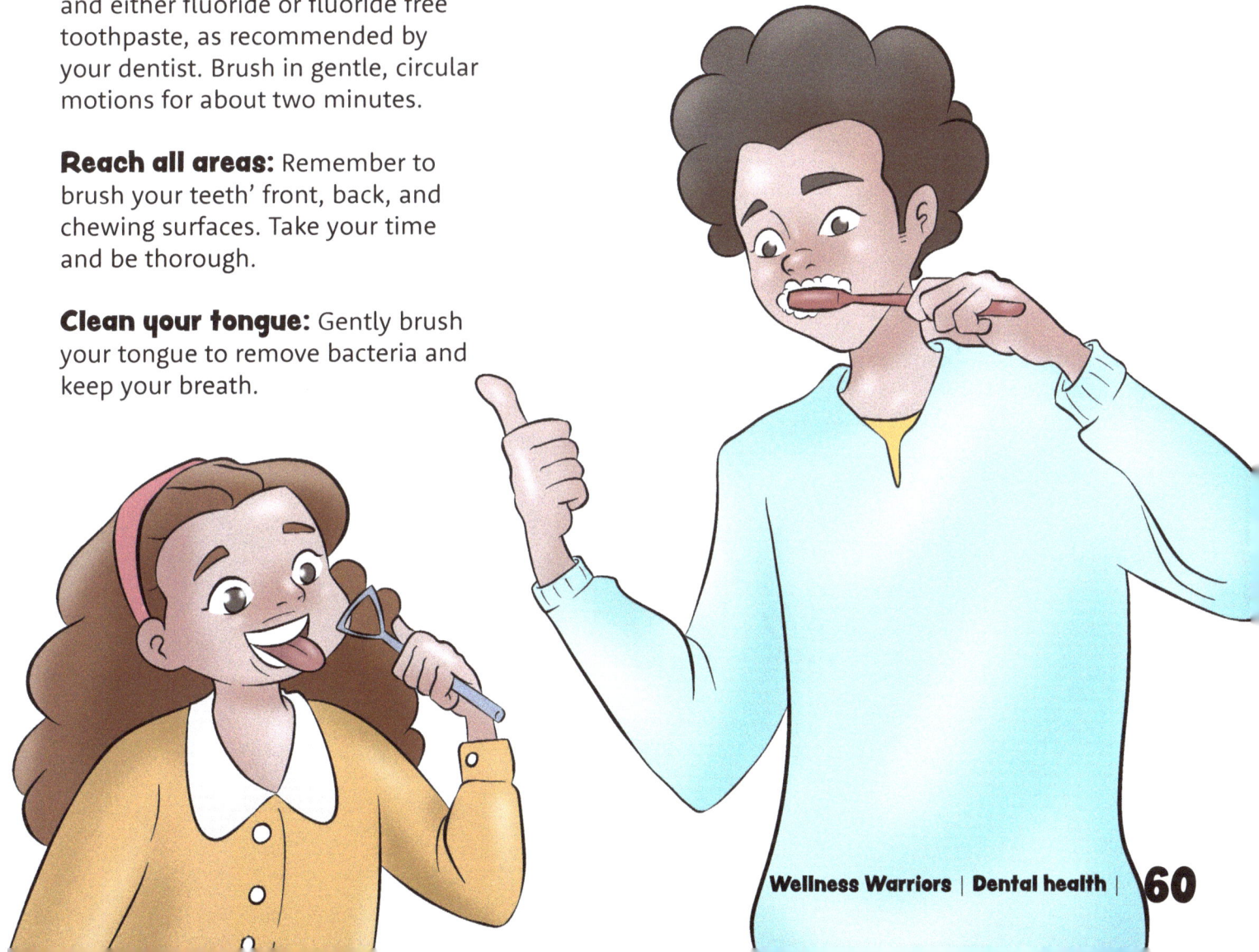

Flossing Fun

Flossing is like a superhero cape for your teeth, reaching where your toothbrush can't. Here's how to do it right:

Use a piece of floss: Take about 18 inches of dental floss and wind it around your fingers. Hold it tightly and glide it between your teeth, moving it up and down gently.

Be gentle: Don't snap the floss into your gums. Curve it around each tooth, making sure to clean the sides.

Floss all your teeth: Remember to floss every tooth, including the ones at the back of your mouth.

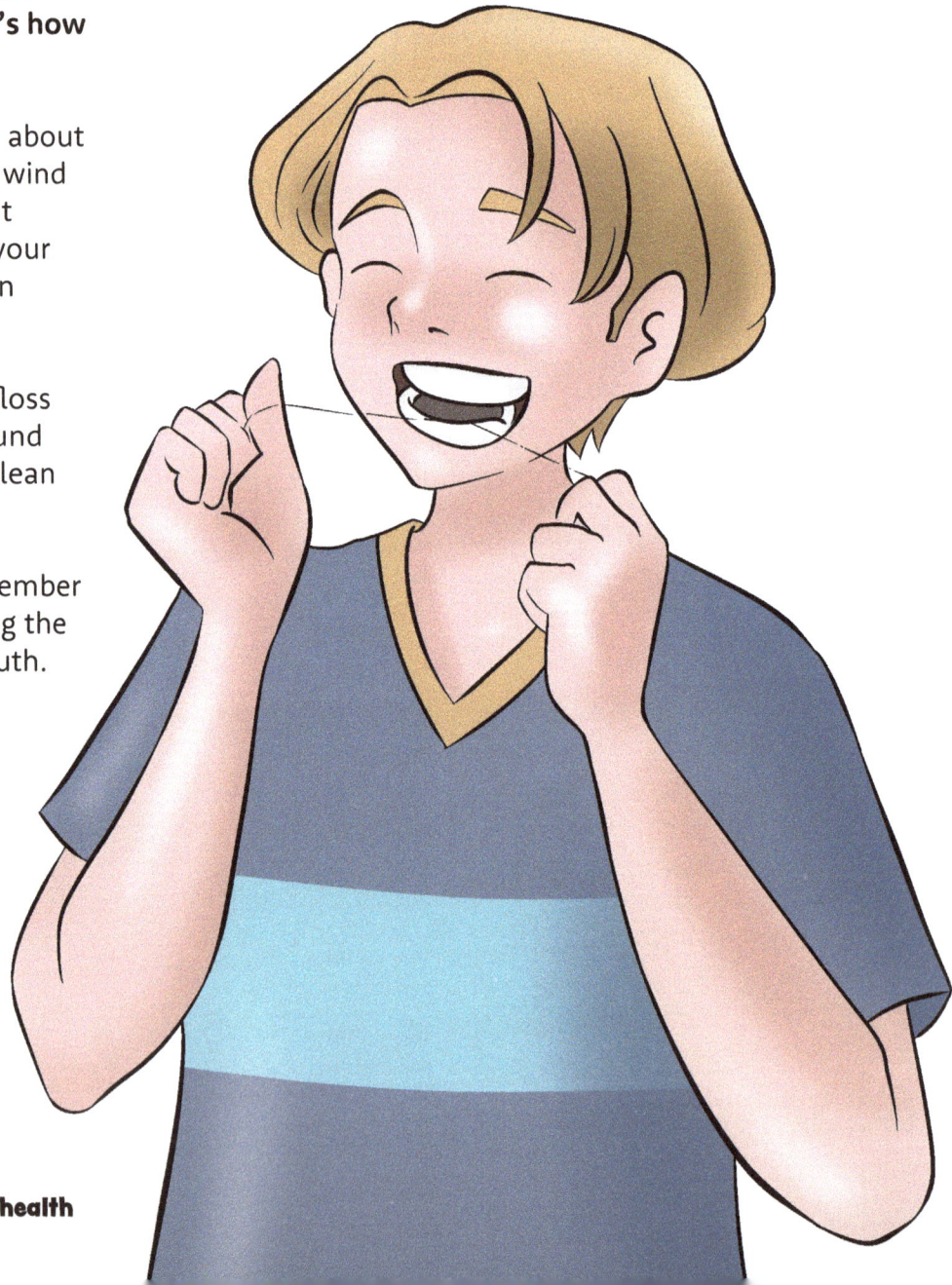

Dentist Visits

Visiting the dentist every six months is crucial for maintaining a healthy smile. Here's why:

Dental check-ups: Your dentist will examine your teeth, clean them, and check for any problems like cavities or gum disease. Don't worry; they're there to help you!

X-rays: Sometimes, the dentist may take X-rays to see if there are any hidden issues in your teeth or jaw.

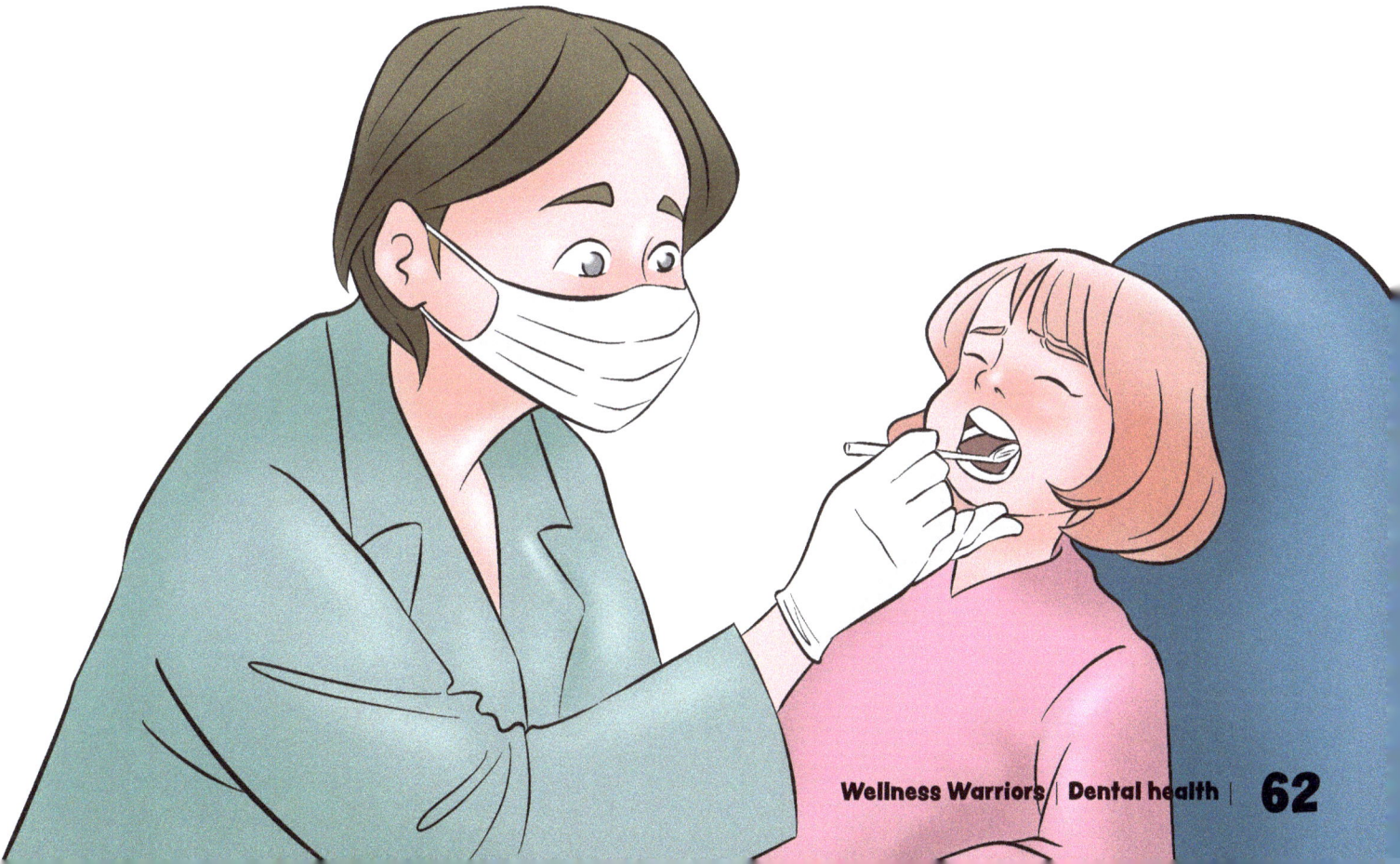

Try It Activities

Brushing challenge:
Set a two-minute timer and brush your teeth using gentle, circular motions. Imagine you're a superhero fighting off evil bacteria!

Flossing race:
Challenge a family member or friend to a flossing race. Who can floss all their teeth correctly and in less time? Ready, set, floss!

Draw your super smile:
Grab some paper and colors. Draw yourself with a bright, healthy smile, showing off those sparkling teeth.

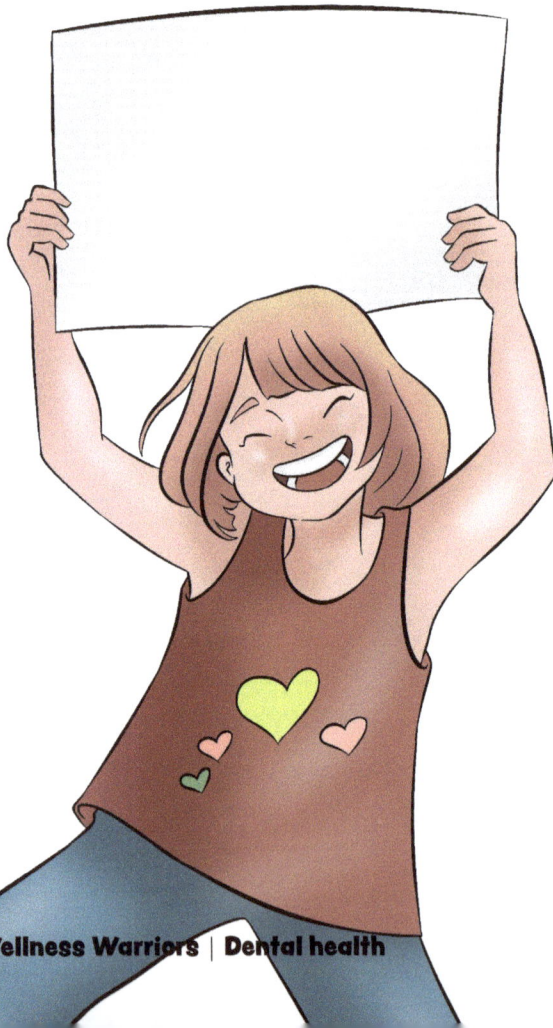

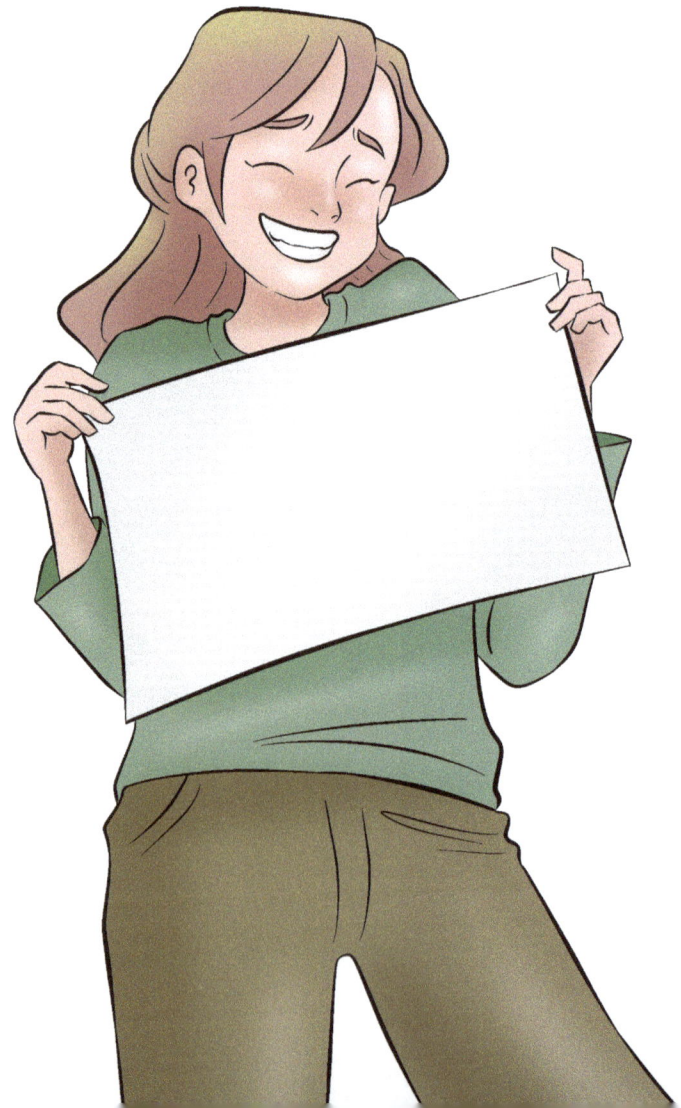

"

Remember, taking care of your teeth is something that you can control. You're keeping your smile healthy and strong by brushing and flossing regularly and visiting the dentist. So, keep up the great work, and let your smile shine bright like a star!

Chapter 9
Mental Health

Did you know your emotions affect your health?
It's true! Taking care of your mental well-being
is as important as your physical health.

Feelings Matter

Emotions are like superpowers that can make you feel happy, sad, excited, or even a little bit scared. Here's what you need to know:

Recognize your feelings:

Pay attention to how you feel throughout the day. Are you happy, angry, worried, or something else? Emotions are like colorful clues that help you understand yourself better.

Express yourself: Find healthy ways to express your emotions. Talk to a trusted adult, draw a picture, write in a journal, or engage in creative activities that help you express what you're feeling.

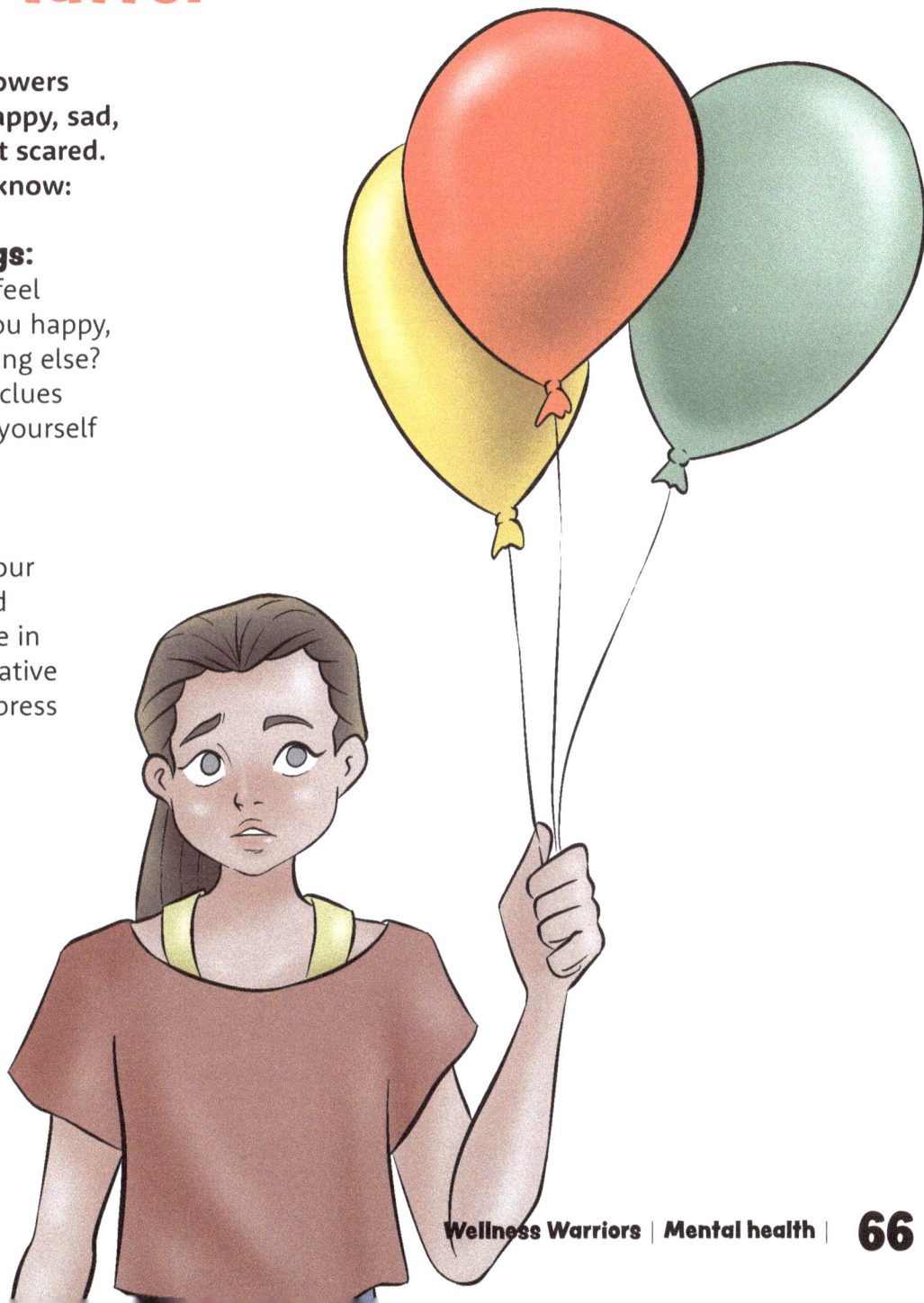

Building a Support Team

Just like superheroes have allies, having a support team is essential for your mental well-being. Here's how to find the right people:

Trusted adults: Talk to your parents, teachers, or other grown-ups you trust about how you're feeling. They can offer guidance, support, and a listening ear.

Friends: Share your emotions with your friends. Sometimes, just talking about how you feel can make a big difference.

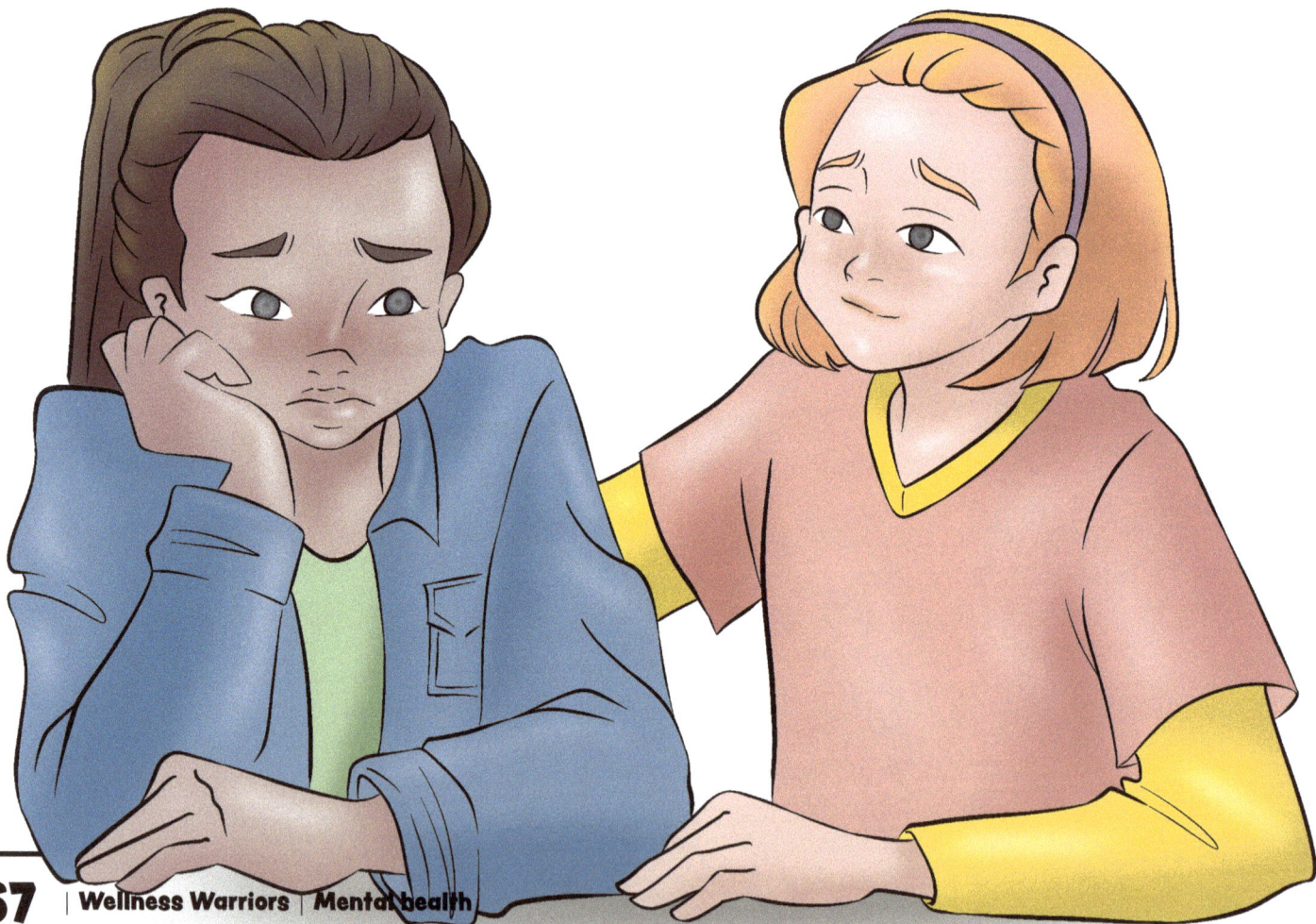

Try It Activities

Engaging in activities that make you feel good is a powerful way to boost your mental health. Here are some activities to try:

Emotion journal:
Create an emotion journal where you can write or draw your feelings daily. How are you feeling? What made you feel that way? How can you make yourself feel better?

Feelings charades:
Play a game of charades with your friends or family, acting out different emotions and guessing what each other is feeling. It's a fun way to explore emotions together.

Create a calm-down corner: Design a cozy space in your room where you can go when you need some quiet time. Fill it with pillows, blankets, and items that make you feel calm and relaxed.

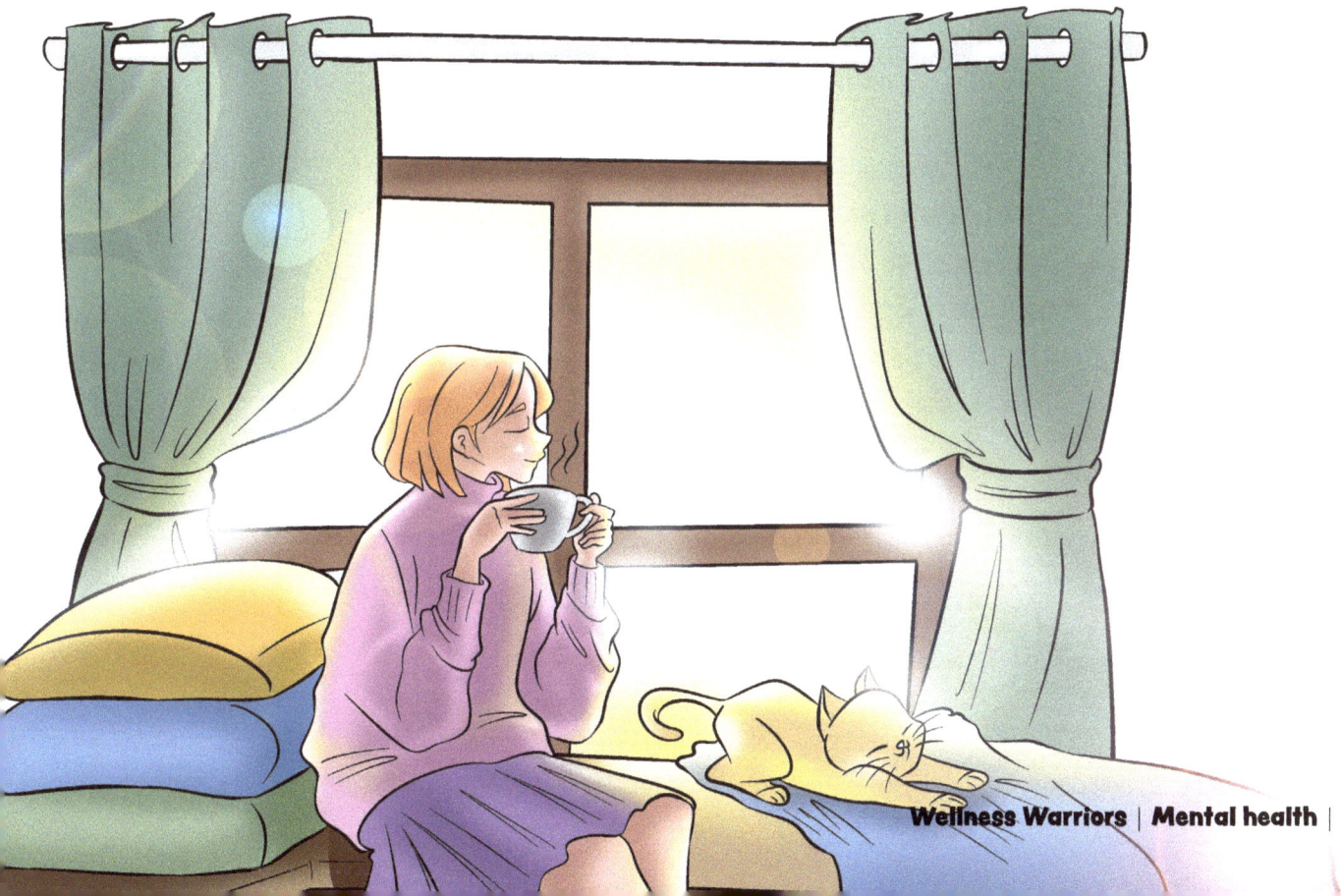

Chapter 10

Rest and Recovery

Did you know that rest is just as important as being active? It's true! Your body needs proper rest to stay strong, avoid injuries, and keep your energy levels at their peak. Are you ready to recharge? Let's dive in!

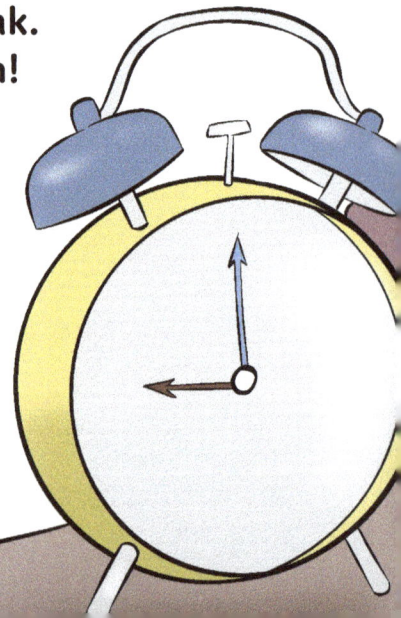

The Power of Zzz's

Sleep is like a magic potion for your body. It helps you grow, boosts your immune system, and keeps your brain sharp. Here's what you need to know:

Bedtime routine: Create a relaxing bedtime routine. Take a warm shower or bath, read a book, listen to calming music, and do not use your phone or other devices an hour or more before bed. Your body and mind will thank you!

Sleep duration: Aim for 8+/- hours of sleep each night. It may sound like a lot, but your body needs that time to rest and recharge.

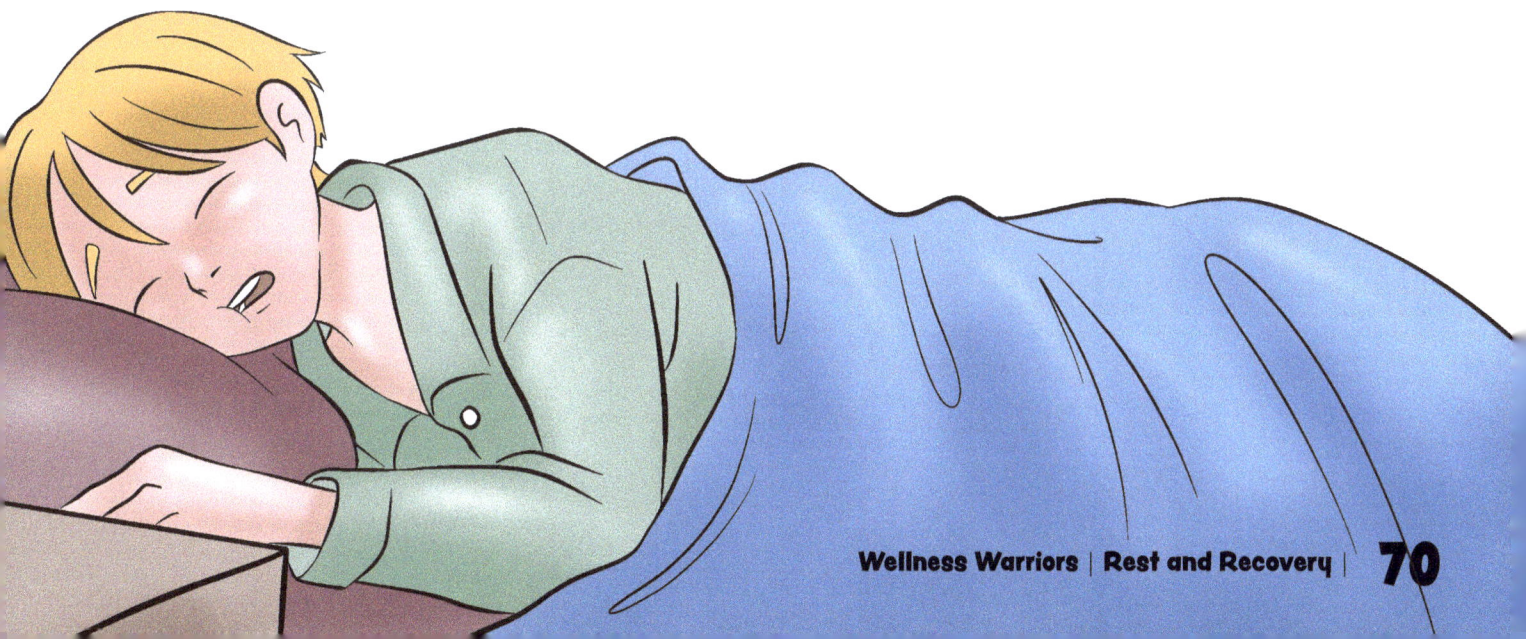

Rest Days are Repair and Building Days

Everyone needs to take breaks. Here's why:

Muscle repair: Intense sports or running activities can strain your muscles. Rest days give them time to repair and become even stronger.

Injury prevention:
Overuse injuries can happen when you don't give your body enough rest. Taking regular breaks helps prevent these injuries and keeps you in top form.

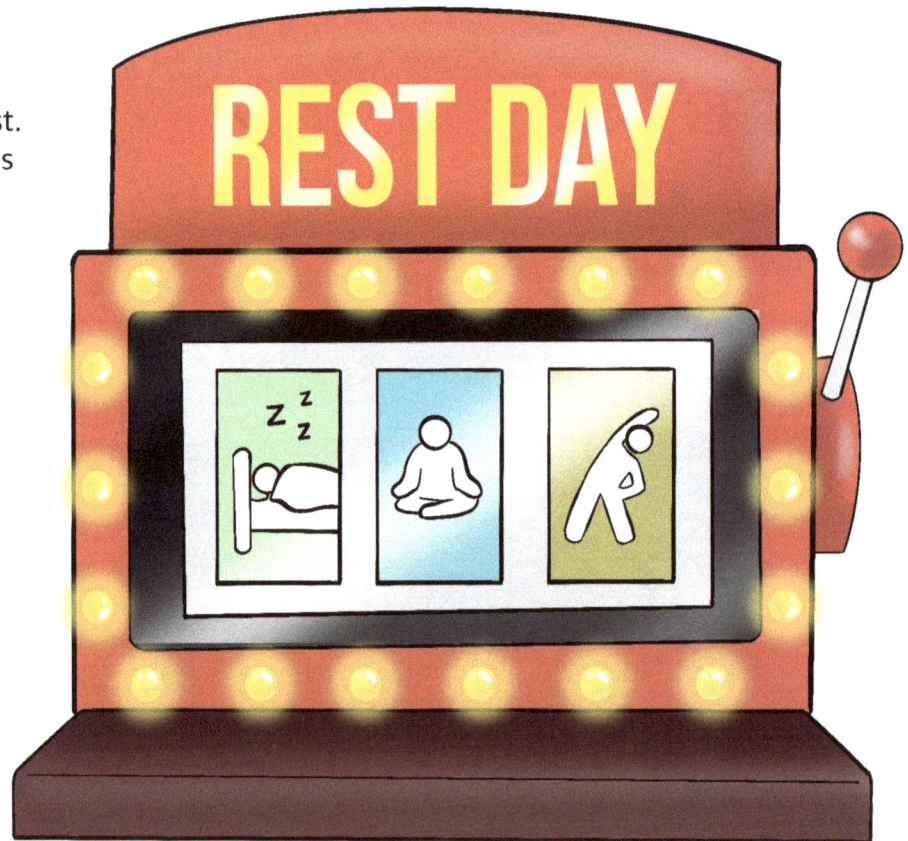

Rejuvenating Activities

During your rest days, engage in activities that help your body recover and rejuvenate. Here are some ideas:

Gentle stretches: Practice gentle stretching exercises to relax your muscles and improve flexibility.

Creative outlets: Engage in activities like drawing, painting, or writing. They allow your mind to unwind and unleash your inner creativity.

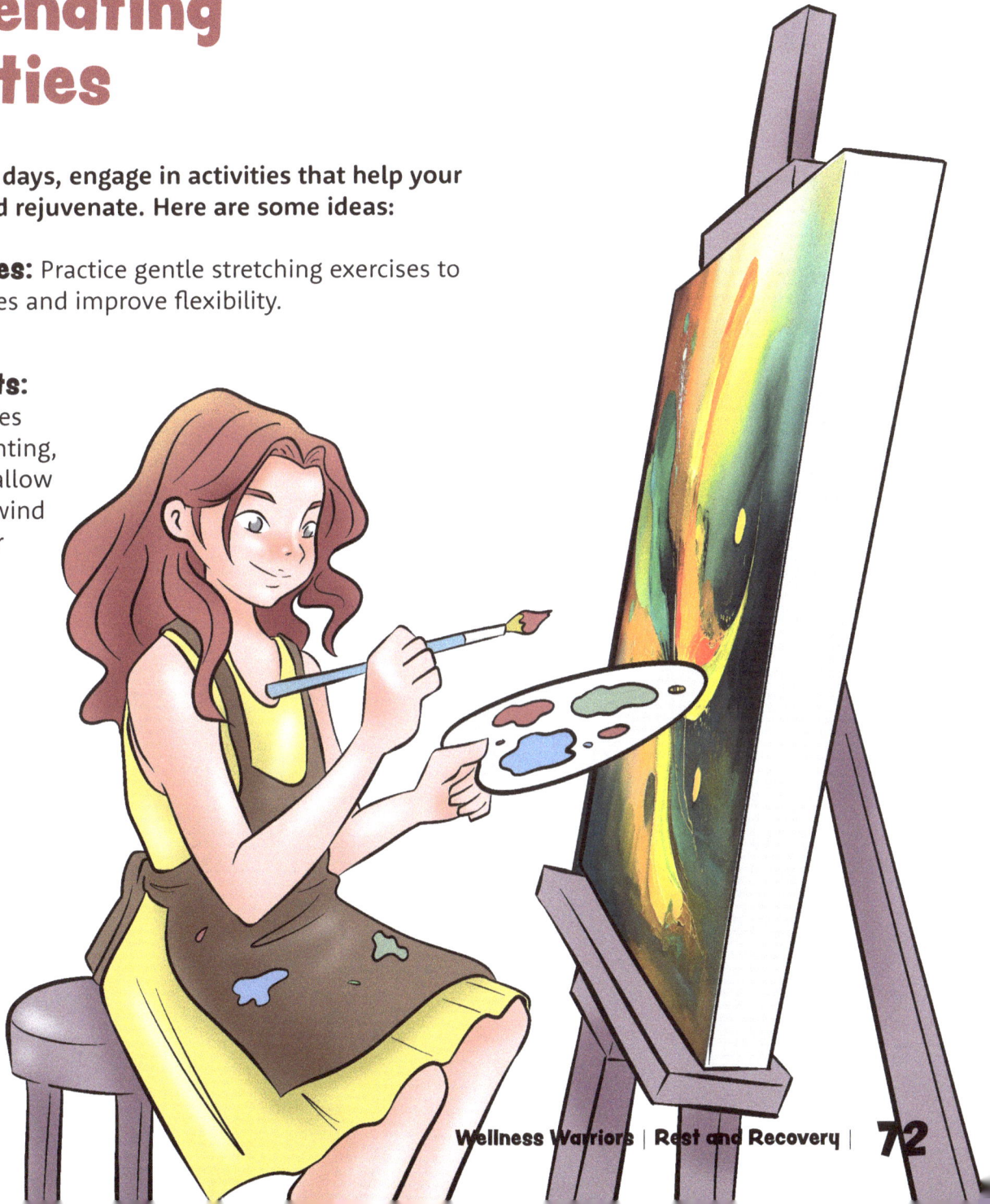

Try It Activities

Sleep log:
Keep a sleep log for a week. Write down what time you go to bed and wake up. How many hours of sleep are you getting? Discuss with your family how you can improve your sleep routine.

Rest and play:
On your rest days, plan activities that involve less intense movement but are still fun. It could be playing board games, solving puzzles, or having a movie marathon with friends or family.

Mindful break:
Take a 5-minute break daily to sit quietly and focus on breathing. Close your eyes, take deep breaths, and let your mind relax. Notice how you feel afterward.

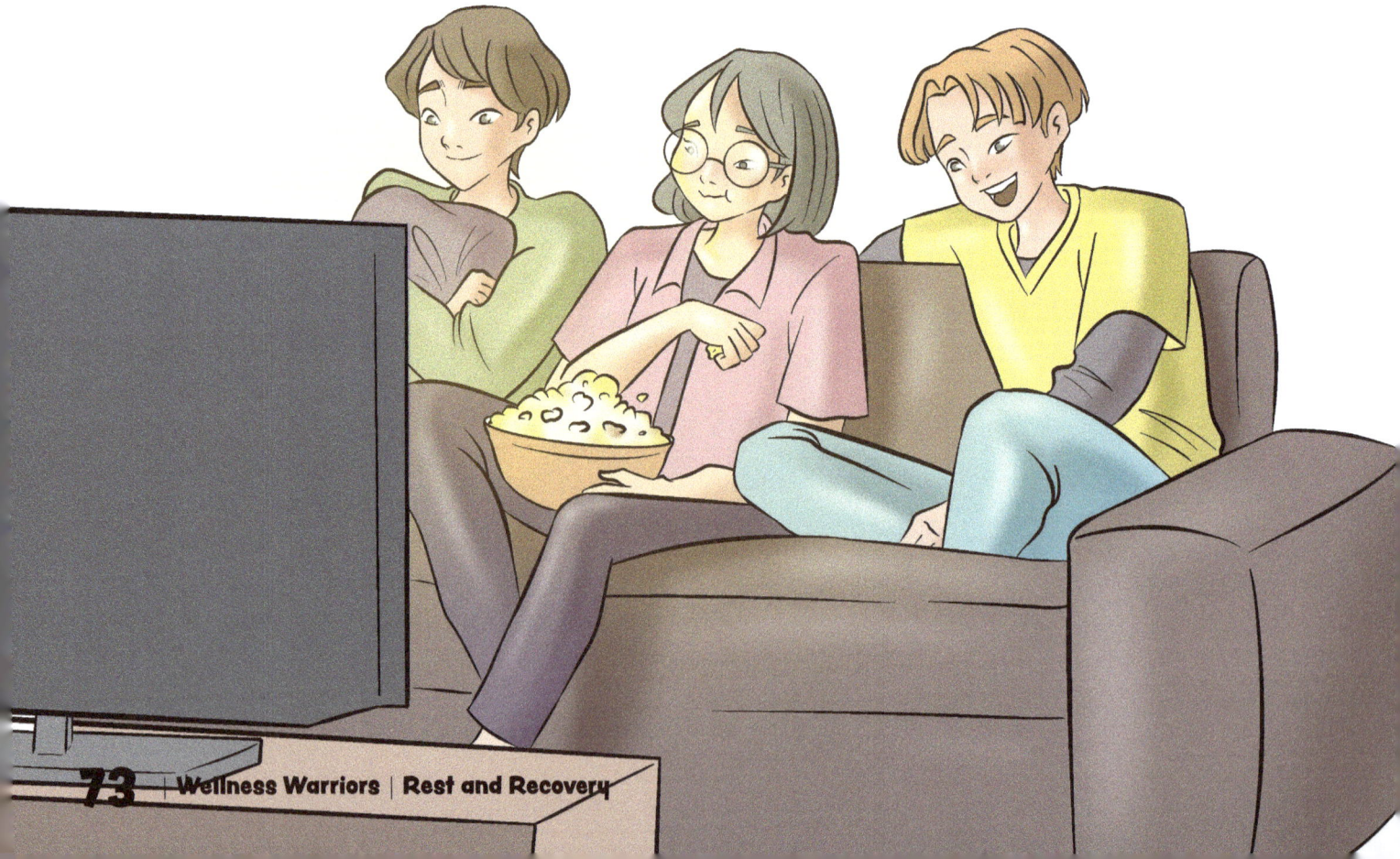

"

Remember, rest and recovery are not signs of weakness but acts of self-care and strength. Getting enough sleep, taking rest days, and engaging in rejuvenating activities gives your body what it needs to stay healthy, strong, and injury-free.

In Closing...

Nicely done Wellness Warriors! You've completed a fantastic journey to a healthier and happier you in this book. We've covered ten important topics that have given you the knowledge and skills to boost your well-being.

But remember, this is just the start of your lifelong journey toward feeling your best. Keep using the exercises and strategies you've learned, and share what you know with others to inspire them on their wellness journey.

Always involve trusted adults in your wellness journey; they can offer guidance and support. Together with your friends, you can create a community of health-conscious people who want to live the most vibrant and fulfilling lives possible.

Outdoor Skills

About The Authors

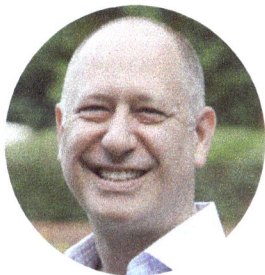

For the past 25 years **Mort Greenberg** has been a salesperson and sales manager for technology start-ups and larger media companies. Fighting his way up from an Account Executive to a role as a division President you can guess there were many challenges that needed to be overcome. Along the way Mort launched two companies, FitAd and MindFlight and learned many hard-fought lessons that start-ups are not always successful. He is a graduate of the State University of New York at New Paltz where he studied International Relations and Economics. While in college he started a company selling screen printing and promotional items to local businesses and on-campus organizations. At the same time, he also volunteered as a Congressional District Intern for the U.S. House of Representatives. He is an Eagle Scout and in junior high school bought several newspaper routes from neighborhood kids to create his first business. Mort is also the author of "Revenue Vs. Sales", a three book series that you can find on Amazon.com

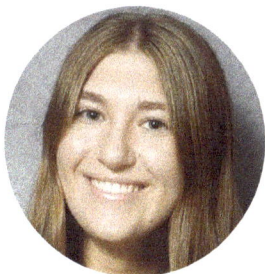

Carly Greenberg attends the University of Maryland's Smith School of Business with a double major in marketing and mana—gement. Carly's twin brother has autism, and she has helped him find his voice through her unique interactions with him. He is the original little guy with greatness. Carly is the original fearless girl, always helping others, volunteering, and finding ways to do more with less - all while having to put up with a crazy dad. Carly also holds a black belt in Tae Kwon Do.

www.ingramcontent.com/pod-product-compliance
Lightning Source LLC
Chambersburg PA
CBHW042340030426
42335CB00030B/3415